Medicine & Society
In America

Medicine & Society In America

Advisory Editor

Charles E. Rosenberg
Professor of History
University of Pennsylvania

ESOTERIC

ANTHROPOLOGY

(THE MYSTERIES OF MAN):

A COMPREHENSIVE AND CONFIDENTIAL TREATISE ON THE
STRUCTURE, FUNCTIONS, PASSIONAL ATTRACTIONS,
AND PERVERSIONS, TRUE AND FALSE PHYSICAL
AND SOCIAL CONDITIONS, AND THE MOST
INTIMATE RELATIONS OF MEN AND
WOMEN

——————

By T. L. NICHOLS, M.D., F.A.S.

*A*RNO *P*RESS & *T*HE *N*EW *Y*ORK *T*IMES

New York   1972

Reprint Edition 1972 by Arno Press Inc.

Reprinted from a copy in
The University of Illinois Library

LC# 75-180585
ISBN 0-405-03962-X

Medicine and Society in America
ISBN for complete set: 0-405-03930-1
See last pages of this volume for titles.

Manufactured in the United States of America

ESOTERIC
ANTHROPOLOGY

(THE MYSTERIES OF MAN):

A COMPREHENSIVE AND CONFIDENTIAL TREATISE ON THE
STRUCTURE, FUNCTIONS, PASSIONAL ATTRACTIONS,
AND PERVERSIONS, TRUE AND FALSE PHYSICAL
AND SOCIAL CONDITIONS, AND THE MOST
INTIMATE RELATIONS OF MEN AND
WOMEN.

———

BY T. L. NICHOLS, M.D., F.A.S.,

Author of "Human Physiology," "The Diet Cure:
Eating to Live," "The Beacon Light," "How
to Live on Sixpence a Day," etc., etc.

———

LONDON:
NICHOLS & CO., 34 HART STREET, W.C.

HAY NISBET & CO. LTD.,
PRINTERS,
73 DUNLOP STREET,
GLASGOW.

TO THE READER.

PREFACE TO THE AMERICAN EDITION.

I HAVE a few words to say in explanation of the motives, plan, and intention of this work; not to the public, but to the individual reader. I have no public to appeal to or propitiate; but only the person who now reads these words. They are written for him or her, and are intended to be *private and confidential.*

This is no book for the centre-table, the library shelf, or the counter of a bookseller. As its name imports, it is a *private treatise* on the most interesting and important subjects. It is of the nature of a STRICTLY CONFIDENTIAL PROFESSIONAL CONSULTATION BETWEEN PHYSICIAN AND PATIENT, in which the latter wishes to know all that can be of use to him, and all that the former is able and willing to teach. It is such a book as I would wish to put into the hands of every man and every woman —yes, and every youth wise enough to profit by its teachings— *and no others.*

Moreover, it is such a book as no one has yet written. We have ponderous works on anatomy, dry details of organism, buried in Greek and Latin technicalities, with no more life than the wired skeletons and dried preparations which they describe. We have elaborate works on physiology, and popular books on the same subject; the former are cumbrous, and incomprehensible to any but a professional reader; the latter are often meagre and shallow, and neither contain a clear philosophy of life and health. Within a few years there have been some earnest works written upon special subjects in physiology and pathology, which have been very useful; but I know of no comprehensive treatise.

The books on some of the most important matters treated of in the following pages, are, for the most part, either the result of an unscientific enthusiasm, leading to great errors, or a morbid pruriency of imagination, or devices of the most unscrupulous quackery. Of this latter class, there are scores of books, each containing a portion of truth, but each full of errors, and each intended to make money directly by their sale, and still more to bring practice in some special line of medical or surgical quackery. It is a distinctive feature of this class of works, that in every few pages will be found a tempting bait for a personal consultation, or a course of treatment. And this is the design of nine-tenths of all the medical books now published.

I write from other motives, and for other purposes. I write, not to get consultations, but to prevent their necessity; not to attract patients, but to keep them away; and to enable them to get health without my further care. I wish to make this book so full, so clear, so thorough, and complete, that every one may understand the structure and functions of his system, the conditions of health, the causes of disease, and all the modes and processes of cure. It is a book for the prevention of disease; for the preservation of health; and, as far as that end can be attained, for its restoration. Having faithfully and carefully written it, I shall have performed a part of my duty. I shall have done the work at once, and for all, instead of wasting my life in a thousand individual efforts. Henceforth, when a patient consults me, I shall say with honest old Abernethy, "Read my book!" I wish, as far as possible, to retire from practice; to devote my remaining years to the more congenial pursuit of education, literature, and social science. But, before I could do this, I felt that I had a great duty to perform. The following pages are the result of my endeavour to perform that duty.

As the material basis of all reform, and all progress of humanity toward its true destiny, the world wants health. Individuals are sick, communities are sick, nations are sick. The very earth is diseased. All must be cured together; but the work must begin with the individual. Every man who purifies and invigorates his own life, does something for the world. Every woman who lives in the conditions of health, and avoids the causes of disease, helps the race; and if such persons combine their purified and invigorated lives in healthy offspring, they do a noble work for the redemption of universal humanity.

My heart glows with the thought that this book will be the means by which thousands of men and women may preserve health for themselves, and transmit it to whole generations of strong, wise, and happy beings; that it may be one of the instrumentalities of a real, physical redemption for mankind, out of which will be developed all moral excellence, intellectual elevation, social harmony, and individual and general happiness.

Its plan and method are the result of long reflection, and a desire to give just what was necessary to the design, and no more. That design is to give, as far as possible, either what does not exist in any other work, what lies buried in a mass of error, or hidden under scientific disguises, or what it is thought necessary to exclude from works intended for general circulation.

Finally, I rely upon the calm judgment of the reader, for whom this volume is prepared, and to whom it is expressly sent, at his or her own desire.

And now, my human brother or sister, all I ask of you is, that, with a clear mind, and a pure heart, a love of the truth, and a willingness to accept it, you read the following pages; and, so far as the teachings they contain commend themselves to your reason, that you follow them faithfully in a life of purity and devotion to the highest good. There are many things which may be contrary to your preconceived notions. Humanity lies prone under the errors of ages. The miseries of mankind are but the symptoms of its errors of thought and life. There is no disease without a cause, and the cause is closely related to the remedy.

The world is cursed by ERROR and DISCORD—it must be saved by TRUTH and LOVE.

PREFACE TO THE ENGLISH EDITION.

In 1853, near New York, in the second year of the American Hydropathic Institute, while giving daily lectures to a class of male and female students on Anatomy, Physiology, and Hydrotherapeutics, I found the need of such a manual of health as I wrote in the following pages, written for those I was then teaching, aided by Mrs. Nichols, some record of whose labours for health may be found in "A Woman's Work in Water Cure and Sanitary Education." This book soon found a very wide circulation. I believe fully a hundred thousand copies have been printed, and it has found its way to the most distant corners of the world. Large numbers have been brought to England.

I received a letter from a missionary in the Fiji Islands, from which I copy a few sentences :—

"I bought 'Esoteric Anthropology' in Sidney when I was preparing to come down to these islands as a missionary, some years ago. That book I have found to be a most excellent companion in this out of the way place, and have many a time thanked you for it. Two years ago, I sent an order to America for another copy, that I might supply a friend with it, and received a new edition, called by a new title, 'The Mysteries of Man.' I am thoroughly satisfied with the book—but there is one point I write to ask you about, in which the last edition differs very materially from the first. In the portion concerning the treatment of natural labour, you say in the new edition :— 'When the delivery is completed, I take the vagina syringe and throw a pint and a half of TEPID water,' &c. Now in the first edition, you recommend COLD water for that purpose, as also does Mrs. Nichols in her Experience [Woman's Work.] This is a very important point, and may mean life or death, I therefore write to ask you.

"Doctors are scarce in Fiji. Nearly two years ago, my wife was confined, and, as I was the doctor, monthly nurse, and everything else, I followed the plan I thought best, and that was the plan of your 'Esoteric Anthropology.' All went on well, and I have spoken of your plan of treatment to my friends. Mrs. Nichols' writings are very valuable, particularly in a place like Fiji."

Naturally I was pleased with this letter, and naturally I was also very indignant at the alteration made in my book without consulting me, since it has passed beyond my control. I wrote to my Fiji friend that the water must be COLD, and I resolved that I would at the earliest possible moment prepare a thoroughly revised edition of my book in England, from which I would expurgate all the errors of twenty years ago, and into which I would put some truths I have learned since it was written.

"Esoteric Anthropology," though covering a portion of the same ground, yet varies widely from my recent work, "Human Physiology the Basis of Sanitary and Social Science." It treats more particularly of disease, and more practically of treatment—especially of the conditions and diseases of the reproductive system, and of gestation and childbirth. "Human Physiology" treats more of Social Science, and three of its six parts are devoted to matters which are but slightly touched in the Anthropology. One may therefore well be the sequel or companion of the other. I have honestly tried to make both of them thoroughly good and useful books, true in science, pure in morals, and containing the principles of the highest welfare of man and of humanity.

T. L. N

CONTENTS.

ILLUSTRATIVE ENGRAVINGS.

———

ESOTERIC ANTHROPOLOGY.

CHAPTER I.

OF MAN AND HIS RELATIONS.

A MAN is an organised being, with the consciousness of existence, and of having certain faculties of thinking, feeling, and acting. By means of his senses, tastes, and attractions, he holds relations to the material universe and to other beings. Each man is the centre of his universe. All things relate to him. He is an egotist, in this sense, by the necessity of his nature. His first idea is of the consciousness of his own existence; and on this first thought all his knowledge depends.

When man studies his own organisation, physical and mental, he finds that he is made with relations of perfect fitness or harmony with nature. The world is full of beauty, and he has eyes adapted to see it, and faculties fitted to enjoy it. His ears are wonderfully adapted to all sounds and their harmonious combinations. His sense of smell is related to a thousand delightful odours. His taste finds exquisite gratification from the aliments best adapted to supply the waste of his system. His pervading sense of touch, modified in many organs, gives him a world of delights. We can realise the uses and pleasures of these senses, only by trying to fancy ourselves deprived of one or more of them.

As the senses, feelings, and faculties of man connect him with the universe, he cannot fail to perceive that his relation with that universe is, or should be, harmonious, and that a beautiful harmony pervades all nature, marking it as a work of design.

From the evident harmonies of man and the universe, comes necessarily the idea of God, as the Creator, pervading intelligence or soul of this universe of matter and thought. And the idea, or belief in God, comes to man as irresistibly as the recognition of his own consciousness. We have thus three things existing: the individual man, the external nature with which he holds harmonious relations, and the Author of these harmonies of relation, and all things between which they subsist; that is, between *all* things; for nature, to be in harmony with man, must be in harmony with itself in all its parts.

Out of the harmony of these relations of God, nature and man, or the individual soul, comes the belief in immortality, which comes directly from a necessary harmony between desire or attraction, and the thing desired; for the eye is no more a proof of light, and the ear of sound, than the "longing after immortality" is a proof of its necessary existence. "Attraction," says a great philosopher, "is in proportion to destiny." God has not mocked man with desires never to be fulfilled, and an ideal never to be realised.

Man desires health, wealth, knowledge, love, happiness; let him only live in harmony with nature, and they are all his—and they can be his only in proportion as he lives in this harmony.

When man obeys the laws of his own being, he lives in harmony with nature.

When man is in harmony with nature, he is in harmony with God, the Author of all harmonies.

For a man to follow nature, to live according to physiological laws, or to obey God, is one and the same thing. In doing one he does the other. "For whether we eat or drink, or whatever we do, let us do all to the glory of God."

The Cause of causes, being infinite, is of necessity incomprehensible. We reason from effects to causes, and form some idea of a maker from what he has made. But we know too little of nature to form any definite or comprehensive idea of the Author of Nature. We know almost nothing of matter or force, or what we call the laws of nature. We do not know how or why a stone falls to the ground, or water runs, or the sun gives light and heat, or life exists on this and probably other planets. The more we know of nature, and especially of ourselves, the better is the idea we are able to form of the power, wisdom, and goodness of the Creator; aside, of course, from such revelation of his character and attributes as he has seen fit to give us.

Man, in his body and his soul, is a revelation of God; and in his developments, sexes, faculties, instincts, passions, and relations, is to be devoutly studied. If we would learn the will of God, we may find it here; but as man is, to a great extent, in a state of discordance with nature, we can only understand him rightly by studying him in his best conditions and most harmonious relations.

The First Cause must be self-existent, and therefore eternal and infinite, filling space and duration. Principles are self-existent. We cannot conceive of any time or place when a circle did not differ from a square, and the three angles of a triangle did not make two right angles.

Fourier, in his analysis of universals, defines the first principles of nature as—

1st. The active principle, or SPIRIT.

2nd. The passive principle, or MATTER.

3rd. The neuter principle, or MATHEMATICS.

Equivalent to God, universe, laws.

In this work, we have to consider man as an organised being, possessing certain faculties and passions, and the relations he sustains, through these, to nature and to his fellow-beings.

Health is the result of the integrity of a good organisation, and the harmony of true relations.

Disease is the consequence of the reverse of both these conditions.

The law of universal analogy connects man with the universe. His life depends upon light, heat, and other elements or forces, generated in the sun, a body nearly a hundred millions of miles distant, but to which man and the earth are so united, that the least change in the centre of the solar system instantly affects every planet, and every thing they contain. Man stands at the apex of the visible creation. In him matter, and force, and life, have their highest expressions, and it is for this reason that human physiology is a central or pivotal science. On it is based a knowledge of God and his laws; the universe and its divine harmonies, man and his destiny, social and individual.

We shall see that the subject of HEALTH relates to all these; that the causes of DISEASE are in the discordances of man and nature, and that the conditions of health belong to the harmonies of the universe.

The fully developed man, of the highest type with which we are acquainted, is a beautiful and majestic animal, six feet high, walking erect on two legs; with an oval-shaped head, balanced upon a perpendicular spinal column; with two arms, furnished with prehensile organs of a curious and complex structure. He has a soft, smooth skin, of a rosy white colour, and fine hair grows upon the head, chin, and around the virile organs.

The female of this animal is commonly shorter than the male, more delicately formed, with longer hair upon the head, and none on the face; with smoothly rounded limbs tapering to smaller hands and feet; with narrower shoulders, wider hips, and a beautiful bosom.

The sexes differ in mental and moral qualities, as much as and corresponding to the differences in bodily organisation. There is sex in mind and soul.

Man is gregarious in his habits, the love of society being one of his strongest instincts. He builds houses and other structures of use and ornament; makes arms, clothing, and means of artificial locomotion; subdues other animals to his service; has an articulate and written language; produces music by his own natural organs, and by instruments he has invented; forms statues and pictures; prepares food by fire, and in a thousand ways shows himself widely different in his nature and faculties, and therefore in his destiny, from all other animals.

Many animals possess remarkable faculties, and several of those we have mentioned as belonging to man. Bees have mathematical skill, some kind of language, great industry, and a limited power of adapting themselves to circumstances. In birds there is often seen great mechanical power, and fervour of feeling. In the mammalia—the dog, the beaver, the horse, and the elephant, we have limited reasoning powers, and some high moral attributes. But all animals have either no power of progress, or a very limited educability. Man alone seems capable of infinite progression, and of an intellectual and moral development of the extent of which we have probably very inadequate conceptions. He alone is free, with choice of good and evil, and therefore moral accountability. His capacity for improvement is a capacity for perversion and depravation. God could not give him the power of progression without also giving him liberty of action; and liberty implies the power of doing wrong. Man could not have had the power of being sublimely great and happy, without the liability to become degraded and miserable. In order to do good, he must have been made at liberty to do evil; and that he might feel the glorious satisfaction of doing right, it was necessary that he should have the dangerous faculty of doing wrong.

But however degraded and depraved man may become, there is no doubt of his immense superiority to all animals; we find his nature more complicated in its details, more numerous in its parts, more exquisite in its formation, and more admirable in its adaptations, than any of the wonders of nature around us. We must compare man with other organised beings, to do full justice to the wisdom and beneficence displayed in his structure, functions, and capabilities for happiness.

Happiness, enjoyment, pleasure, or whatever word may express our sense of the natural and harmonious action and gratification of the human passions, appears to be the single end or final cause of creation. We are unable to conceive of any other motive. Every faculty is for use, every organ has its function, and every function gives, or in some way contributes to, enjoyment. Nothing is made in vain. Every thing in man and out of him, is the result of infinite wisdom, joined to an infinite love; and therefore all tends to one single purpose, the greatest possible happiness of all beings.

We are to study the organisation of man, therefore, with a constant reference to its adaptation to happy uses, and we shall find that he has no organ, structure, or tissue, which is not marked with the design of a great artist, who had a special and benevolent motive in making man, and the wisdom and power to accomplish that design. In this study, we cannot go one step without faith in God, and an acceptance of His manifestation to our consciousness. Every one must accept what commends itself to his reason as true, or in harmony with his conscious being.

When we contemplate any phenomenon, we wish to understand the cause. "What does it?" is a spontaneous question. This inquiry of causation leads directly to the cognition of the Great Cause of causes.

CHAPTER II.

THE CHEMISTRY OF MAN.

I WISH to make a few observations on the chemistry of man, before entering upon his physiology.

As a material being, man is subject to the laws of matter. Fire burns his body, acid corrodes it, and when, in the language of poetry, "the vital spark has fled," this matter becomes subject to the processes of putrefactive decomposition. The matter of which the body is composed returns to its primitive elements, or enters into new forms of organic matter.

Chemistry treats of the elements of matter, and their relations, combinations, and changes. An elementary body is one which the chemists have not been able to separate into simpler elements. There are now reckoned over fifty of these elements, all but a few being metals, and many found in small quantities, and having, so far as we now know, but little importance. The most important so-called elementary bodies—for chemists do not despair of resolving many of them into simpler forms—are iron, copper, gold, silver, zinc, tin, mercury, etc., among the metals; aluminum, potassium, sodium, calcium, silicon, etc., among the metallic bases of the earths and alkalies; oxygen, hydrogen, nitrogen, chlorine, etc., among the gases; and carbon, sulphur, phosphorus, etc., among the peculiar bodies, not otherwise classified.

The metals found in the human body are—*iron*, which gives its colour to blood; *sodium*, which, united with chlorine, forms common salt; *potassium*, which exists in minute quantities as potash; *calcium*, the metallic basis of lime, which forms the hard structure of bones and teeth; and *magnesium, silicon*, the basis of sand, rock crystal; *alluminum*, the basis of clay, slate, etc., and some other metals are sometimes found in minute quantities.

Oxygen is one of the most important and univer sally diffused of all the elements. It composes one-fifth of the atmosphere; one-third by measure, and seven-eighths by weight of water, and combines with metals and other elements, to form a vast variety of substances. Some of these combinations are called oxides, some acids, some alkalies. Oxygen is the chief supporter of combustion, which is but another name for oxydation. This process is accompanied by the evolution of heat, and, under some circumstances, of light. It is the grand element of all organic life, and is believed to be the chief agent in all vital operations.

Hydrogen is the lightest of the gases, and combines with oxygen to form water. As water is a large component of all organised bodies, and pervades earth and the atmosphere, we have in nature an abundant supply of hydrogen. United with oxygen, it produces flame, and the result of such union is water.

Nitrogen forms four-fifths of the atmosphere, and is an important constituent of vegetable and animal tissues, helping to form albumen and fibrin, both vegetable and animal. United with hydrogen, it forms ammonia; combined with oxygen, chemically, it forms nitric acid.

Carbon exists in nature, as charcoal, mineral coal, and is crystallised in the diamond. It is the chief constituent of woody fibre, oil, starch, sugar, alcohol, and enters largely into all vegetable and animal substances. Combining with oxygen, it forms carbonic acid gas— a heavy irrespirable fluid, in which men drown, as if under water. Carbon is constantly separated from the blood by the lungs, liver, and skin. Combining with oxygen, it furnishes animal heat, and the result is car-

bonic acid. Hence the necessity for constant ventilation. Carbonic acid is also produced by fires, the
burning of lamps or candles, and in most cases in
which carbon combines with oxygen. The result of
their rapid union is the disengagement of intense light
and heat.

Sulphur is a peculiar and familiar substance, which
unites readily with oxygen, burns, and forms sulphuric
acid. It is found in vegetables, and is thence carried
into the blood and muscular tissues of animals. From
the combination of sulphur and oxygen (sulphuric acid)
with various bases, we have the sulphates of soda,
magnesia, iron, zinc, etc.

Phosphorus is something like sulphur, but much
more inflammable—that is, it unites more readily with
oxygen at low temperatures. In this union it forms
phosphoric acid. This combines with calcium, and
forms phosphate of lime ; and this, existing in wheat
and other vegetables, makes part of the blood of animals, and is found especially in the bones.

All matter, whether solid, liquid, or gaseous, is composed of ultimate atoms, inconceivably minute, as the
microscope everywhere reveals to us ; as the smallest
animalcule is composed of parts formed from a combination of a vast multitude of such atoms. These
atoms have their own determinate form, size, weight,
motions, attractions, repulsions, and peculiar powers
of whatever kind.

Two or more atoms of simple elements uniting, according to laws of definite proportions, form the molecule
of the composed body. Thus, one atom of oxygen,
uniting with one atom of hydrogen, forms one molecule
of water, and they can only so unite in these fixed proportions. One atom of nitrogen, uniting with five
atoms of oxygen, forms nitric acid, and so on.

No two atoms of matter can ever, by any possibility,
come in contact with each other. This is a fact which

I have not space here to prove, but which is perfectly demonstrable. No two atoms of diamond, or gold, or water, or air, ever can touch each other. They are held in a certain nearness by their attractions, but forever kept asunder by their repulsions. Each one is an independent individual atom, but holding social relations with the atoms around it.

The distances of these atoms from each other, and their relative positions, change continually with variations of temperature. Thus, a hard body expands and contracts with every variation of heat and cold—that is, each of its atoms goes farther from or approaches nearer to its neighbours. With the increase of heat, their repulsion increases, until they break apart, and the solid becomes a liquid; with a still further increase of temperature, the liquid becomes a vapour.

The same kinds of elementary atoms may combine in the same proportions, producing various results, depending, not upon their nature or proportions, but upon some form of combination. Thus, the fœtid gas from the gas-works, and the beautiful perfume, otto of roses, are composed of exactly the same elements, combined in exactly the same proportions. The ingenious reader will soon be surprised to find how nearly alike are the chemical ingredients of all animal substances.

All forms of matter exist in virtue of certain laws, under which they maintain their conditions and identities. As long as certain attractions and repulsions exist, in a certain relation of intensity, there is no change; but change conditions, and the atoms instantly assume new relations and new forms. With the simple addition of caloric, ice becomes water, and water steam; with the abstraction of caloric, steam is condensed to water, and water solidifies. Under a similar rise of temperature, the solid substance gunpowder, or gun-cotton, assumes instantly a gaseous form, and the added repulsion of its atoms acts with tremendous and destructive force.

So, if we bring the element of electricity, in the form of galvanism, to act upon water, we disturb the attractions of the atoms of oxygen and hydrogen for each other. The oxygen obeys a stronger attraction, and goes to one pole of the battery, while hydrogen rises from the other. And such, in some way, is the condition of all compositions and decompositions; and similar laws, founded on a system of universal analogy, run through the whole universe of matter and of mind. Every atom of matter, and every human soul, left in freedom, follows its strongest attraction.

Of the great number of substances reckoned elementary, many enter into the complex combinations of the organic world, but there are only a few which seem necessary. The rest are occasional or accidental. Thus, in the vegetable kingdom, we have carbon, oxygen, hydrogen, and, in less quantities, nitrogen. The three first are the principal constituents, the fourth is always present; and a variety of others, as soda, potash, lime, iron, sulphur, phosphorus, etc., may be present in varying proportions.

Animals are made up of the elements existing in vegetables. There is no other source except the two compound elements, air and water. Man can only have what these can give him. In all the phenomena around us, we have only changes of form and relation. Men consume the flesh of animals, but this is only taking vegetable elements at second hand.

The proximate constituents of the animal body are divided into two classes, the *mineral* and *organic*.

We may divide the mineral into the physically useful, the chemically useful, and the merely incidental.

The constituents useful by their physical properties are:

   1. Water, composed of hydrogen and oxygen, and

which is, therefore, an oxide of hydrogen; and if hydrogen be considered a metal, water is a mineral. Water constitutes about nine-tenths of the body by weight. It pervades every tissue. A beefsteak, as it comes from the market, contains about 70 per cent. of water. The blood and nervous matter are nearly all water. Man begins his existence as a microscopic vesicle of almost pure and transparent water.

2. Phosphate of lime comes next to water among the mineral constituents of our bodies, in quantity and use. It forms most of the solid matter of bone, and is found also in blood, from which the bone is made, in milk, and also in the urine and fœces, by which its waste and surplus is expelled.

3. Carbonate of lime, which forms the shells of fish, snails, etc., is also found in small proportions in the bones of the higher animals and man.

4. Phosphate of magnesia also unites with the phosphate of lime, though in minute proportions.

Of chemically useful constituents, we have:

1. Hydrochloric acid, one of the constituents of common salt, from which it is obtained, in the digestive fluid.

2. Chloride of sodium, or common salt, in the blood, gastric juice, bone, urine, tears.

3. Carbonate of soda, found in animal ashes.

4. Phosphate of soda, in blood, lymph, bile, etc.

5. Iron in the colouring matter of blood, hair, black pigment of the eye, etc.

The incidental constituents are chloride of potassium, alkaline sulphates, carbonate of magnesia, manganese, silica, allumina, arsenic, copper, mercury, lead, etc.

The organic constituents are divided into two groups; those which contain nitrogen, and those which are destitute of that element.

Protein is a name given to the nitrogenised substance which, under various forms, enters into the composition of the most important animal tissues. It is albumen in the white of an egg, in the serum of the blood, and many of the secretions; fibrine in the fibrous portion of the blood, in membrane, muscle, and areolar tissue; and casein in milk. All these are composed of the same ultimate elements, viz., carbon, oxygen, hydrogen, and nitrogen, united in the same proportions.

Fibrine, casein, and albumen, all exist in vegetables, and are identically the same in them as in the animal tissues. So far as nutrition is concerned, it makes no difference whether we eat vegetable food or animal, only that it is purest at first hand, while the flesh of animals is always more or less tainted with disease or diseasing impurities.

The same ultimate elements enter into the composition of gelatine, the basis of bones, cartilages, sinew, ligament, skin, etc., and the chemical bases of saliva, the gastric juice, bile, and are found in pus, urine, and other excretions.

The animal sugars, fats, and acids are composed of carbon, oxygen, and hydrogen, but contain no nitrogen. They differ but slightly from similar vegetable productions.

As the blood contains all the proximate principles that enter into the human body, its analysis will show of what that body is composed.

Healthy human blood contains, in 1000 parts :

Water	790·0	Cruorin†	1·0
Fibrine	0·9	Carbonate of soda	1·0
Albumen	54·0	Chloride of sodium (salt)	4·0
Hæmatin*	133·4	Chloride of potassium	2·0
Oxide of iron	0·7	Phosphates of lime and	
Phosphorised fat	8·2	magnesia	0·5
	Carbonate of lime	1·3	

The blood also contains sulphur, phosphorus, and

---

* Colouring matter of the blood globules.
† A protein compound resulting from albumen and fibrin.

occasionally several other substances not given in this analysis.

Human milk, being secreted from the blood, and again converted into it, gives a similar result. In 1000 parts:

Water.......... ..... 883·6 | Casein (cheese) .... 34·3
Butter .... 25·3 | Sugar of milk, etc....... 48·1
Salts........ 2·3

Cow's milk, the most commonly used for food, may be compared with the above by the following analysis. In 1000 parts:

Water................ 821·8 | Casein................ 67·0
Butter .... 55·0 | Sugar, etc............. 51·0
Salts, etc......... 13·0

The atomic composition of the proteian compounds albumen, fibrine, and casein, is carbon, 40; hydrogen, 31; nitrogen, 5; oxygen, 12; or by Liebig's formulary, C 48, H 36, N 6, O 14.

Crystals of the sugar of milk contain carbon, 12; hydrogen, 12; oxygen, 12.

The animal fats and acids are composed of these three elements, as are the vegetable oils, starch, sugar, and acids.

By certain changes in the arrangement of the atoms, and sometimes in their proportions, we have starch converted into sugar, fat, alcohol, acid. Sugar is converted readily into fat by the digestive process, and into alcohol and acid by fermentation.

Thus we have the three elements, carbon, hydrogen, and oxygen, composing the heat-giving principles, in our food, and nitrogen added to form the animal tissues.

Much of what is stated here will seem more clear and important, when it is applied to physiology, in what is to follow.

CHAPTER III.

HUMAN ANATOMY.

THE human body, viewed outwardly, is composed of a head, neck, trunk, two superior extremities, and two inferior. Standing before you, facing, or the reverse, a line down the centre divides it into two equal and symmetrical portions. This is the case with the body, as a whole, but is not the fact respecting the internal organs, which are not symmetrical, or cannot be divided into two equal halves. But the bones are either symmetrical, or in pairs, and so are all the muscles of the system of voluntary and instinctive motion.

The trunk contains three cavities: the upper, the chest or thorax; the middle, the abdomen; and the lower, the pelvis. The thorax contains the heart and lungs; the abdomen contains the stomach, intestines, liver, spleen, pancreas, kidneys; the pelvis contains the bladder, rectum, the ovaries, uterus, and vagina in women, and the seminal vesicles and prostate gland in men. In the latter, the most important generative organs are external.

The head is divided into two parts; the face, which forms a small angle of its anterior inferior portion, and the cranium, an oval box of bone, filled with the brain, a prolongation of which extends about three fourths of the length of the back-bone, or vertebral column, and branches or fibres from which are sent off to every part of the body.

The whole body is made up of several systems of organs or tissues, which enter into every part of its structure. Thus we have—

1. A bony skeleton, or frame-work of two hundred and forty bones, with their cartilages and ligaments, giving it form, solidity, and power of motion.

2. A muscular system, consisting of four hundred muscles with their tendons, by which all motions are performed, and extending over the whole system make a large portion of its bulk.

3. An areolar or cellular system, composed of fine interwoven fibres, making the sheaths of vessels, muscles, nerves, and forming the parenchyma, or connecting substance of various organs. It is in, or upon this tissue, that the fat cells are deposited.

4. The arterial system, by which the blood is carried from the heart to every part of the system, supplying bones, muscles, nerves, skin, membrane, etc., with the vital fluid which sustains them all, and repairs their hourly waste. The ramifications of the arteries are inconceivably minute. The point of the finest needle pierces hundreds of blood-tubes, the moment it penetrates the true skin.

5. And wherever the blood is carried by the arteries, it must return by the veins; so that we have a venous system, as vast and pervading as the arterial.

6. A portion of the blood, believed to be the finest and most highly vitalised, is returned to the heart, from every part of the system, by another system of vessels, or tubes, called lymphatics; these form a net-work over the whole body, and penetrate to every part of it.

7. The nervous matter connected with the brain, is also distributed to every part of the system, so that the needle which draws blood by piercing microscopic veins and arteries, also gives exquisite pain, by wounding the delicate fibres of the nerves of sensation.

8. As the nerves of the ganglionic system, called nerves of organic life, accompany the blood-vessels in their minutest ramifications, these nerves must equally pervade the whole organisation.

Here, then, we have eight pervading systems, each of which extends to the entire body, and most of which would preserve its entire and perfect form, if deprived of all the others.

Among the extensive and important tissues of the human body, we must not omit the external skin, which lines the whole surface of the body; the internal skin, or mucous membrane, which lines its interior parts, which are connected with external apertures; and the serous membranes, which line the shut cavities, and are folded around the most important organs.

All these tissues and organs we must briefly consider.

Bone is composed of nearly equal parts of cartilage (gristle) and earthy matter. The cartilage is first formed, and then the earthy matter is deposited. Each is deposited by the blood, which contains in itself the materials of every tissue and every secretion. Bone is an organised, living structure, pierced by blood-vessels and nerves, subject to waste, and requiring renewal, liable to fracture and disease, and demanding reparation. Seemingly solid, it is very porous, so that a piece of bone has been compared to a heap of empty boxes, thrown loosely together.

Bones are long, as the arm and thigh bones; cuboidal, as those of the wrist and instep; or flat, as the shoulder-blades and skull bones. They are joined closely and immovably, by sutures, or a sort of dove-tailing; by symphisis, as in cartilaginous joinings; or by movable joints, as those of the shoulder and hip. There are ball and socket-joints, allowing the bone to be moved in all directions, as the thigh and shoulder joints, while the elbow, knee, ankle, and other joints are called hinge-joints, allowing only of the simple movements of flexion and extension.

The ends of the bones have a covering of cartilage, and the joints are firmly bound together, and curiously strengthened by ligaments. If the best artist or mechanician in the world were to exert his ingenuity a thousand years, he could discover no better method of making a skeleton.

The bony structure of the head is very complicated. There are eight bones in the cranium, and fourteen in the face. The former are mostly flat, and inclose the brain, to which they offer an admirable protection ; the latter are of various irregular shapes, forming the nose, jaws, orbit of the eye, roof of the mouth, etc.

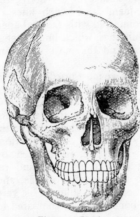

Fig. 1.—Cranium.

The head rests on the spinal column, which is composed of seven cervical, or neck vertebræ, twelve dorsal, or back, and five lumbar, or those of the lower part of the back. This column, which increases in size from above downward, rests, at its base, upon the sacrum, a wedge-like bone which forms the keystone of an arch, made by the bones of the pelvis, which, in their turn, rest upon the thigh-bones, and these again on the bones of the legs and feet. Twelve ribs on each side are attached to the dorsal vertebræ; these curve round in front, and by cartilaginous connections with the sternum or breast-bone, form the bony case of the thorax, and protect the heart and lungs. The arms are joined to the body loosely, by means of movable shoulder-blades, which are kept in place by muscles, and by means of the collar-bone.

The points about the bony skeleton most worthy of notice, are:

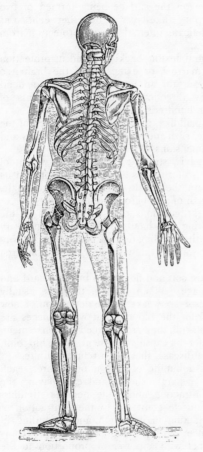

Fig. 2.---Full Length Figure showing Bony Skeleton.

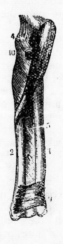

Fig. 3.---Pronators of the Fore-Arm.

The protection of the brain by the eight bones of the cranium; those on the surface being formed of two plates with a sponge-like layer of bone between, so as to give the delicate internal organs protection from external injuries.

The strong and flexible backbone, and its protection of the spinal marrow, or extension of the brain; so formed as to sustain an immense weight, to bend easily in every direction, and to afford points of attachment for hundreds of muscles.

The coat-of-mail-like, movable thorax, formed of the dorsal vertebræ, ribs, and sternum, which expands and contracts in dimensions in rising and falling.

The bony pelvis, strong to support the weight of the body, and so formed as to sustain and protect its contents; and in the female larger than in the male, to allow the birth of a full-grown fœtus.

The rolling articulations of the two bones of the fore-arm, allowing the hand to be turned in every direction, and the combination of small bones, forming the flexible joint of the wrist, and the flexible arch of the foot.

The bones are soft and flexible in infancy, hard and brittle in old age. When broken, they are usually repaired in five or six weeks by the deposition of new bony matter from the blood. But where pieces are taken from the skull, they are replaced by dense membrane; and under the capsular ligament, at the hip joint, and in states of disease, they often refuse to unite.

A muscle is a bundle of very minute fibres, each contained in a separate sheath, and each having the property of contracting under the nervous stimulus As the whole muscle contracts, by the contraction of its fibres, contracting in its length, and expanding in its circumference, it draws the parts to which it is attached together with a power in proportion to the size of the muscle and the stimulating force applied.

The nervous power has, in fact, more to do with the force exerted than the strength of the muscle; and the force of contraction is often much greater than its own power of cohesion. The contraction or drawing together of the particles or disks, of which the ultimate fibres of a muscle are composed, under the nervous influence, resembles the development of the magnetic attraction in pieces of iron under the galvanic current.

The sheaths of the muscular fibres seem to unite together, to form the tendons by which they act on distant parts, when compactness is wanted for use and beauty, as in the wrist and ankle.

The head alone has seventy-seven muscles. There are eight for the eyes and eyelids. The eyeball has four straight muscles, one above, below, and on each side, and two oblique, to give it a rolling motion. One of these, before it is attached to the eye, passes

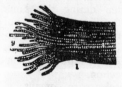 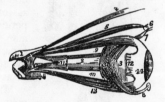

Fig. 4.—Muscular Fibre, dividing into fibrillæ, magnified 300 diameters.

Fig. 5.—Muscles of the Eyeball, from outer side of right orbit.

through a pulley, to change the direction of its action. There are eight muscles for the lips, eight for the jaw, eleven for the tongue, seventeen for the motions of the head and neck; and it is by the variously combined action of these that we have all our movements and expressions. There are seventeen muscles for the movements of the chest, abdomen, and loins. These perform, among others, the important function of res piration. The cavity of the chest is enlarged some eighteen times a minute, by raising the ribs and sternum, and still more by straightening or drawing down the

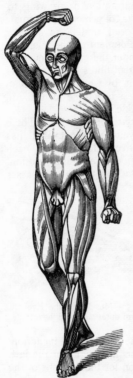

diaphragm, or muscular separation between the thorax and abdomen. When this is done, the air rushes into the lungs, to prevent the vacuum that would otherwise be formed. Next, the three sheets of abdominal muscles contract, force up the diaphragm, draw down the ribs, and forcibly expel the air: and this action is kept up, night and day, sleeping and waking, from the moment of birth till death; while the heart, a muscular organ, contracts four times as often during the same period. The whole body of man, in all its parts and organs, is, during all this time, the scene of various and constant action.

Muscles are organs of voluntary or involuntary, conscious or unconscious, motion. We have no direct control over the heart, or the muscular fibres of the stomach, intestines, bladder, uterus. We can govern some-

Fig. 6.—Muscular System.   what those of respiration. The muscles of swallowing are involuntary. When a morsel of food is pressed back by the tongue beyond the fauces, it is seized, and by a series of involuntary contractions, carried into the stomach.

The largest and strongest muscles are the extensors of the lower extremities, and the flexors of the upper. Thus we have large masses of muscle on the back of the leg, forming the calf, to extend the foot; on the front of the thigh, to straighten the knee-joint, and again on the posterior portion of the pelvis, to extend the thigh. Much of the beauty of the human form depends upon this muscular arrangement.

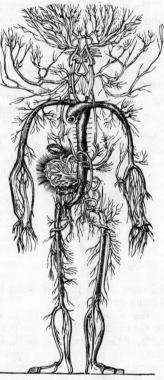

Fig. 7.—Arterial System.

The bones and muscles give form and locomotion, and the whole body is a means for the manifestation and enjoyment of the soul, whose especial organ is the brain. This brain, in which resides the conscious ME, the individual, is carried about, protected, nourished, and variously ministered to by its bodily organs, to which, in turn, it distributes vital energies. In dis-

case, there is discordance between brain and body--
in insanity, the discord is in the brain.

OF THE BLOOD VESSELS.

The necessity for the constant nourishment of the
whole body, growing out of a constant waste of matter
by its activity, makes needful a vast system of tubes
by which the blood may be carried everywhere, and
returned again to the centre of circulation.

We have in the centre of the thorax a heart, consisting of two parts, right and left, each having two

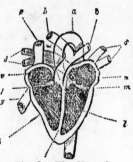

Fig. 8.—The Heart.*

cavities, an auricle and
ventricle. The heart is
simply two force-pumps,
joined together for con-
venience. In some of
the lower animals, as
fishes, there is but a
single pump—in reptiles,
there are three chambers.
Each pump is furnished
with beautiful valves,
which allow the current
of blood to go on, but
prevent its return. These
valves work constantly
for more than a hundred years in some cases, without
getting out of order.

The blood, as it comes from all parts of the system,
by the veins, is received into the right auricle, or receptacle, of the heart, from which, by a muscular contraction, it is sent into the right ventricle. The right
ventricle contracts, and throws the blood it contains

---

* Ideal section of mammalian heart. *a*, arch of aorta; *b*, *b′*,
pulmonary arteries; *c*, superior vena cava; *d*, *d′*, pulmonary
veins; *e*, right auricle; *f*, tricuspid valves; *g*, inferior vena cava;
h, right ventricle; *i*, septum ventriculorum; *k*, descending aorta;
l, left ventricle; *m*, mitral valve; *n*, left auricle.

through the pulmonary artery into the lungs, where it is purified and changed in its colour and qualities. This is the action of the right pump. The blood now goes back by the pulmonary veins to the *left* auricle, thence into the left ventricle; which, contracting, forces it into the great aorta, and so on over the whole body. These two pumps act together. Two auricles contract, then the two ventricles; one pump supplies the lungs, and one the whole body. The right, or lung pump, receives the blood from the body; the left, or body pump, receives it from the lungs.

As there are about twenty-five pounds of blood in the body, and as the heart sends on about **two ounces at** each pulsation, at the rate of say seventy a minute, it is easy to estimate the time it takes for the whole quantity to circulate. But some portions, having farther to go than others, must get round slower. The living blood is the pabulum of life to all parts of the system. It is constantly distributing their substance to bone, muscle, brain, nerve, etc., constantly sending off secretions and excretions, and it must also receive regularly new supplies of matter, prepared from our food, by the processes of digestion. How important that this blood be pure! that our food be natural, and our digestion well performed!

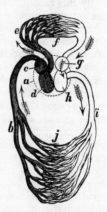

Fig. 9.—Circulation.*

* Ideal view of the course of the circulation. *a*, incloses the four chambers of the heart; *b*, veins bringing dark blood to *c*, right auricle; *d*, right ventricle; *e*, pulmonary artery; *f*, beginning of pulmonary vein conveying the arterialized blood to *g*, left auricle; *h*, left ventricle; *i*, arteries. The arrows show the direction of the current.

From the great aorta which curves over the heart, and then passes down, near the spine, go off branches to the head and brain, the arms, the internal organs, the lower extremities—in a word, to every portion of the body. These branch off, finer and finer, until at last we come to a system of capillaries, or hair-like tubes, of such extreme minuteness, that they can only be seen by microscopes of the highest powers—so fine, that the red globules of blood, which are only the five thousandth part of an inch in diameter, can no longer pass through them, and only the smaller white globules, and finally, the liquid serum alone can find admission.

By this means, blood is everywhere supplied, in just the quantity required. We have it when we want it, where we want it, and as much as we want. In sensitive and active organs, there are many and large arteries, and abundant capillaries, and the supply is active. Thus, four large arteries go to the brain, which receives a large portion, not all. But the heart, a beautiful mechanical contrivance—the most perfect of forcing-pumps—can only send the blood, with a certain force, estimated at fifty pounds, into the main artery. It cannot influence the distribution to one of its branches. It can send it faster or slower, and with more force or less; but this is all. It cannot send blood where it is specially wanted. It cannot send it one hour to the brain, producing active thought and vivid emotions, and the next hour to the stomach, to aid in digestion, and the next to the organs of generation. The heart does not direct the blood to the pregnant uterus, to nourish the growing germ, nor to the broken leg, to furnish a supply of bony matter.

For all this, some other power is needed; a power guided by intelligence, a power which acts upon the nervous system, and which is intimately related to the power of life. Who can comprehend this power which resides in vegetables, in all animals, and supremely in man?

As the blood is sent with a vigorous impetus, from the left ventricle of the heart, through a system of dense, tough, cylindrical tubes, called arteries, over the whole body, by the branchings and ramifications of these vessels, and the networks they everywhere form with each other, until the great branching tree or vine expands to millions of twigs and hair-line tubes of microscopic fineness; so, in order that this same blood may be carried back to the heart, there must be other sets of minute tubes, venous radicles, gradually uniting and enlarging, until the blood is poured through two great tubes, ascending and descending, into the right auricle. Both arteries and veins have the power of expansion and contraction, and do expand to accommodate

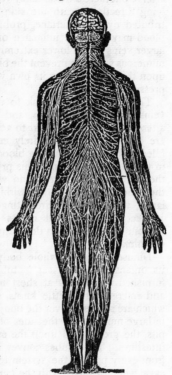

Fig. 10.—Nervous System.

unusual quantities of blood, and do contract, to force their contents onward to their destination. The large

veins generally follow the course of the arteries. In
many parts, there are two veins accompanying one
artery; but there are also many veins which are external,
lying directly beneath the skin, and they are so distributed over the surface, probably, that the venous
blood may have the influence of air and light. The
larger veins in the lower extremities are provided with
numerous valves, to prevent the blood being forced back
upon the capillaries by its own weight, or by muscular
pressure.

The blood is sent back to the heart through the
veins, by capillary action, and this action continues
after the heart has ceased to act, so that the arteries
are commonly found entirely emptied of blood, and
filled with air, while all the blood in the body is found
in the distended veins. This proves that the action of
the heart has no more to do with the circulation of
the blood than to throw it within reach of the capillaries, which have a circulating power of their own.
In fact, trees and all plants circulate their juices
without a heart, and so do many of the lower orders
of animals.

Diffused over the whole body, and penetrating all
its organs, is a third set of tubes, small, transparent,
furnished with valves at short intervals, and entering
and emerging from little knots, or ganglia, or glands,
which are scattered over the body, but which are found,
in large numbers, on the sides of the neck, in the armpits, the groins, and upon the mesenteric folds of the
intestines. These tubes convey white blood, or lymph,
from every part of the system to the descending vena
cava, where it mixes with the current of venous blood,
returning to the heart.

But the lymphatics of the intestines are called lacteals, and convey a portion of the nutriment elaborated
by digestion through the thoracic duct to the same
destination. The anatomy of these vessels has been

but lately understood, and their physiology is little known.

THE BRAIN AND NERVES.

The hollow of the skull, from the top of the head down to a line formed by the base of the orbit of the eye, the opening of the ear, and the top of the back of the neck, and in its entire breadth, is completely filled with a pulpy mass, grey without, and of a pearly white within, called the brain. It is divided into a large ante-

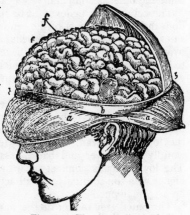

Fig. 11.—The Brain Exposed.

rior and superior portion, the cerebrum, and a smaller pos-terior and inferior portion, called the cerebellum; in the centre, between these, a pro-longation of the brain, con-taining fibres from both, passes down into the hollow of the vertebral column. The por-tion within the skull is the medulla oblongata; the re-mainder is the spinal cord.

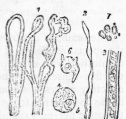

Fig. 12.—Minute Nervous Structure.

It is about half an inch in diameter, and, like the brain, is composed of both grey and white matter, and its different parts have distinct functions. Brain and spinal cord are divided into two equal halves by the median line, so that all its organs and nerves are in pairs, and one side may be diseased or paralyzed while the other is comparatively healthy and active.

The cerebrum is believed to be the organ of sensation, thought, and most of the sentiments and propensities or passions. The cerebellum seems to preside over muscular motion, and is believed by phrenologists to be the organ of amativeness which presides over the generative function. The propensities or instincts, which we possess in common with the lower animals, are found in the lower portion of the brain; the higher faculties, and those peculiar to man, are found in the upper portion. Generally the forehead is intellectual; the top of the head, moral and religious; the side, worldly; the lower and back, passional and selfish. The lower organs connect us with the physical, the higher with the spiritual; and all acting together make up a harmonious being.

The outer grey matter of the brain is composed of cells of microscopic minuteness; the white matter consists of tubes, filled with a still softer substance. All these cells, tubes, etc., are of inconceivable minuteness.

The brain, as the true centre of conscious life, and the special residence of the soul, holds constant communication with every part of the body, and through the five senses with the external world. A pair of olfactory nerves, distributed over the lining membrane of the nose, carries to the brain an impression of odours; the optic nerves, expanded upon the internal chamber of the eye, are impressed with pictures of objects; the auditory nerve, curiously extended through the apparatus of hearing, receives and conveys impressions of sound; the gustatory nerves give us all ideas of savours; and nerves of sensation or touch go off to every portion of the body, especially to the whole surface and its

more sensitive portions. Nerves of motion are also
sent off in pairs from the brain and spinal cord to every
muscle in the body.

The distribution of nervous fibres is as minute as that
of the blood-vessels; and if we reckon the nerves of
organic life, it is much more so. Yet the nerves are
everywhere nourished by the blood, as the blood is
everywhere controlled by the nerves. Blood is formed
under the nervous influence, and nerve matter is continually furnished by the blood. Which is first? If
either, it is the highest, the nerve. The spinal cord is
the first part seen; the brain expands at the end of the
spinal cord.

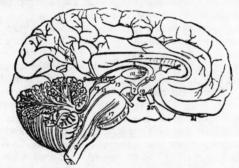

Fig. 13.—Longitudinal Section of the Brain.
Inner surface of left hemisphere and divided cerebellum, showing
the arbor vitæ.

The spinal cord, and brain, and blood are formed
under the influence of nerve matter belonging to the
system of nerves of organic life, called the ganglionic
or sympathetic system.

THE ALIMENTARY SYSTEM.

All organised beings require food. A rock is formed
by a simple, more or less regular, aggregation of atoms,

and there it remains, without change, except as it is acted upon by external agencies. But a vegetable or an animal has an internal growth or development, and is subject to continual changes of form and matter. Every action is accompanied by waste. Each thought, each motion, necessitates a chemical change, by which matter is made unfit to remain longer in the system, or, at least, in the same relations. The waste or effete matter is constantly thrown off in various ways, and new matter must be brought in to fill its place. Vegetables gather this matter from the earth, by their roots, and from the atmosphere by their bark and leaves. Animals obtain their nutriment from vegetables, water, air. In animals the stomach, intestines, lungs, skin, etc., correspond to the roots, leaves, and bark of trees.

Digestion of food begins in the mouth, where it is cut, crushed, and ground by a set of thirty-two teeth, which, in man, differ from those of carnivorous and herbivorous animals, and are adapted to the mastication of fruit, nuts, seeds, and roots. As food is mashed into a pulp by the teeth, it is moistened by the saliva, a digestive fluid, which is secreted from the blood by three sets of glands—the parotid, around the ear; the submaxillary, beneath the angle of the jaw; and the sublingual, under the tongue. When the food is sufficiently mashed and moistened, as it always should be, and mixed with the saliva, which is very necessary to its proper digestion, it is pressed back by the tongue into the pharynx, a membraneous and muscular pouch, which forms the upper part of the throat. The opening of the windpipe is closed by a valve, over which the food passes in safety, and the contraction of the pharynx, and the esophagus, as the narrower portion of the tube is called, force it down through the thorax into the stomach, which is an expansion of this tube, lying a little to the left, below the diaphragm.

When the food has been acted upon by the gastric

juice, which is secreted by the glands of the stomacn, and has been rolled about and churned by the con

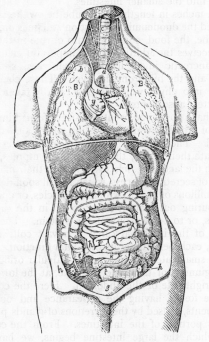

Fig 14.—Vital System.＊

＊ **A.** Heart. **B, B.** Lungs. **C.** Liver. **D.** Stomach. **E.** Spleen. ***m, m.*** Kidneys. ***g.*** Bladder. ***d*** is the diaphragm which forms the partition between the thorax and abdomen. Under the latter is the cardiac orifice of the stomach, and at the right extremity, or pit of the stomach, is the pyloric orifice, below are the large and small intestines. ***i.*** Uterus. ***h, h.*** Ovaries. ***g*** Bladder.

traction of its muscular coats, a portion of it, already prepared to enter the circulation, is absorbed by the veins, as is the water we drink, alcohol, and other liquids, while the remainder passes through the pyloric orifice into the smaller intestines.

Ten inches in length of the tube below the stomach is called the duodenum. Digestion still goes on, and in this tube, the food, converted into chyme in the stomach, receives the addition of two important elements—the pancreatic juice, from the pancreas, similar to saliva, and the bile from the liver. These change the chyme into chyle, which is now rapidly taken up by the lacteal absorbents.

We have now some twenty-five feet of small intestine, in all of which several interesting operations are performed. The veins are taking up such matter as can penetrate their coats; the villi, or little nipples, which contain the lacteal vessels, are selecting their matter by a kind of secreting process, which I shall soon describe; while millions of glands, with their follicles, or openings, are pouring out matter, either to aid in the digestive process, or to be cast out of the system. The entire length of the intestinal canal is a vast collection of organs, each performing its own vital function.

The small intestines open, by a valvular orifice, into the beginning of the large intestine, at the lower part of the right side of the abdomen. Here the contents become fœcal, having the appearance and odour of excrements, caused by the secretions of glands peculiar to this portion of the intestines. From the cœcum with which the large intestine begins, we have the ascending colon, passing up on the right side, the transverse colon crossing over, a little above the navel, and the descending colon passing down on the left side, when it turns backward, and becomes the rectum, terminating at the anus, where a strong round muscle keeps a tight grasp of this extremity of the digestive apparatus. Of the matter taken into the mouth, in a healthy state of the digestive organs, very little finds its way out at the anus. The bran of wheat, the skin and seeds of fruit, woody fibre, and other indigestible matter, is mixed with a much larger quantity of excrement, made up of waste matter of the system, poured into this canal by millions of glands, which separate it from the blood. This is evident from the fact that there may be copious evacuations from the bowels day after day, when no food has been taken.

The intestines are everywhere enveloped by a thin, shining, serous membrane, called the peritoneum, which also lines the sides of the abdomen, and covers its viscera; and they are gathered in their length to a kind of ruffle, called, in its different parts, the mesentery, mesocolon, and mesorectum. In the mesentery and mesocolon are found the arteries that supply the intestines, with the veins, nerves, lacteals, and lacteal glands.

THE LUNGS.

The entire cavity of the thorax, excepting the space occupied by the heart, large blood-vessels, and esophagus, is completely filled by the lungs. They are of nearly the same structure in birds and mammalia, as in man, a spongy mass, made up of air-tubes, air-cells, and blood-vessels, all bound together by cellular tissue.

The windpipe consists of the larynx, or organ of the voice, in the upper and most prominent part of the throat, which opens from the pharynx, just back of the root of the tongue; the trachea, a tube three or four inches long, made up of cylindrical rings and strong membrane, and its branches, or bronchiæ; which fork off to the right and left lung, and afterward divide like the branches of a tree, and are covered with masses of air-cells, into which they open, and which are clustered upon them like leaves on a tree, or more like grapes on a stem; the cells on each twig opening into each other. There are many millions of these cells, and the internal surface of the air-tubes and cells in the lungs is estimated at 150 square feet, or ten times the

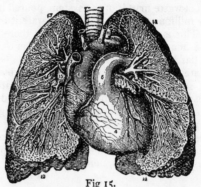

Fig 15.
Heart and Lungs, showing Blood and Air Vessels.

surface of the body. Around each of these minute cells is a network of arterial and venous capillaries, and it is through the coats of these that the air acts upon the blood, giving it oxygen, and receiving from it carbon. There enters, then, into the structure of the lungs, the pleura, or external membrane; the air-tubes and vesicles; the arteries, veins, lymphatics, nerves, and the areolar tissue, which holds them all together.

All the blood passes through the lungs, to be brought into contact with the atmosphere; the animal membranes forming no barrier to the chemical action of gases. This contact of the air with the circulating fluids is necessary to all organised beings—to vegetables and animals. In vegetables this contact takes place in the leaves, in fishes by the gills, in the higher animals by lungs.

THE LIVER.

The size of an organ is *some* measure of its importance. The liver is an irregular-shaped brown mass,
weighing four pounds in health, but often much enlarged in disease. It lies on the right side of the
abdomen, under the diaphragm, opposite the stomach,
and partly covered by the short ribs. The liver is a
collection of a vast number of glands, which separate
the bile from the blood. The blood thus purified is
the venous blood gathered from the stomach and
intestines, which contains a portion of the newly
absorbed nutritive matter. All these veins gather
into one common vein, the vena porta, which enters
and branches out in the liver into minute vessels; the
purified blood collects in another set, and goes to the
ascending vena cava. The gall bladder is attached to
the liver, and serves for a reservoir for the bile, until
it is needed in the process of digestion.

THE SPLEEN.

This is a large glandular organ, situated at the left of
the stomach. It has no excre-
tory duct, no known secretion,
and its function is not understood. It is conjectured to
be a large lymphatic gland.
It is liable to inflammation,
and to enlarging and hardening in malarious diseases.

THE KIDNEYS.

These are hard bodies, of
a flattened oval shape, lying
on each side of the spine near
the last ribs. Each kidney is
a collection of tubes and glands,
ending in a central cavity,

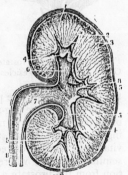

Fig. 16.—Vertical Section
of the Left Kidney.

which opens into long tubes, called ureters. The office of the kidneys is to separate from the blood the urine, which is conveyed by the ureters to the bladder.

The separation of the urine, or rather the solid matter it contains, from the blood is so important that certain death attends its suspension for a short period.

BLADDER AND URETHRA.

The bladder is a membranous and muscular pouch, resting against the pubes in the middle, anterior por-

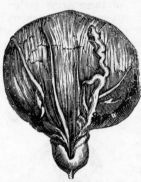

tion of the pelvis. It terminates below in a tube, called the urethra, through which the urine is discharged. In men, the urethra is eight or nine inches long, when at its full extent. In women, it is not more than two inches. The urine is retained in the bladder by a sphincter muscle at its neck.

MALE ORGANS OF GENERATION.

Fig. 17.—Bladder, Prostate Gland, and Seminal Vesicles.

These consist of the testicles, or sperm - preparing organs, the seminal vesicles, the prostate gland, the penis, and their appendages.

The testicles are egg-shaped glands, each consisting of several hundreds of minute, convoluted tubes, ending in a single vessel, which conveys the semen, or vitalising fluid, secreted by these organs, into the seminal vesicles, where it is mingled with a secretion from the prostate gland, and is held in readiness to be ejected through the urethra during the sexual orgasm.

The testicles, in an early stage of fœtal development, are formed close by the kidneys, and gradually
descend to the lower part of the
abdomen, where they pass through
the inguinal canal, and are lodged
in the scrotum. They are sometimes retained in the body.

The prostate gland is a small
body about the size and shape of
a chesnut, just beneath, and partly
surrounding, the neck of the bladder. See Fig. 17. Its secretion seems to be a vehicle for the
semen.

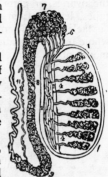

The penis is small in infancy,
and attains at puberty to a length
of from five to seven inches, and
is about five inches in circumference. Its shape is that of a
cylinder, not perfectly regular,

Fig. 18.—Anatomy of
the Testes.

with a soft, delicate cushion, called the glans penis,
at the end. This is the most sensitive portion of the
organ, and in the sexual orgasm is the seat of exquisite pleasure. A soft skin loosely covers the organ,
moveable, and forming a fold, so as partly, and in some
cases wholly, to cover the glans penis.

The internal structure is very curious. In repose,
it is small, soft, flabby, and easily compressible; but
when in vigorous erection, it is distended, hard, and
unbending. The change from one state to the other
occurs in a moment—at a thought or a touch. The
process by which this change is accomplished is not well
understood, but it is probable that the arteries expand
and are filled with blood, while a nervous action con-
stringes the venous capillaries, so that it cannot return.
But all the mechanism and operations of these organs is
very wonderful, and much of it quite incomprehensible.

FEMALE ORGANS OF GENERATION.

These are mostly within the pelvis, and consist of the ovaries, or germ preparing organs ; the fallopian tubes, leading from the ovaries to the uterus, or receptacle of the germ, where it remains during the whole term of gestation ; the vagina, or passage to the mouth of the womb, which receives the penis during

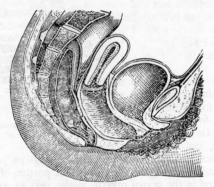

Fig. 19.—Section of Female Pelvis.

the sexual congress ; and the lesser and greater lips and clitoris, a very sensitive organ, resembling the penis, and situated above the entrance of the vagina. The mons veneris is a cushion of fat covered with curling hair, and conveniently placed upon the pubes.

The most important of these organs are the ovaries—egg-formers—of which there are two, one on each side of the uterus, about the size and shape of the testes of the male, and performing a corresponding function. In them are formed the ova, or germs of new beings. When the germ has been perfected its sac bursts with considerable force, it is set free, seized by the finger-like extremities of one of the fallopian tubes, through which it is carried into the uterus.

The uterus is situated centrally in the pelvis, behind the bladder, before the rectum, and four or five inches

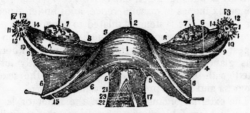

Fig. 20.—Uterus, Ovaries, Fallopian Tubes, etc.

from the mouth of the vagina. It is of a flattened egg or pear shape, with the small end, its neck, downward, and, except in pregnancy, about two and a half inches long. Its mouth can be felt at the upper extremity of the vagina.

In its healthy, unimpregnated state, the walls of the uterus are about half-an-inch in thickness, muscular and vascular, and the cavity is scarcely larger than a kidney-bean. After impregnation it expands so as to contain a fœtus weighing, in some cases, fourteen pounds, with membranes, afterbirth, and fluid weighing as much more. In cases of twins, where there are two fully formed fœtuses and two placentas, the bulk is greater. The uterus expands rapidly, and its minute and imperceptible arteries acquire great size; but in a few hours after birth, it contracts to nearly its previous dimensions. The vagina is a membranous canal, with muscular fibres, lined with a delicate mucous membrane, and forming the passage from the vulva, or external opening, to the uterus. It performs three offices: it allows of the periodical flow of the men-

strual fluid, and the passage of unfecundated germs;
it admits the penis in sexual union, grasping it closely,
and contributing to and partaking of the orgasm; and,
finally, it admits of the passage of the fully-formed
fœtus at birth. Thus a canal, which will sometimes
scarcely admit the finger, expands to receive an organ
five or six inches in circumference, and, under a peculiar action of the system, is dilated to allow of the passage of the head of an infant, which is five inches in its
largest diameter. The vagina is furnished with numerous glands, and, when healthy, is abundantly lubricated with a fluid like saliva, both in the sexual
congress and in the process of parturition.

The external organs consist of the inner or lesser
lips, which are folds of the mucous membrane, called
nymphæ, which seem to shelter and guard the entrance
to the vagina, and the greater or external lips, which
are thicker, and filled with fat, and which close over
the inner. In most cases there is in virgins a thin
fold of membrane, called the hymen, partially closing
the mouth of the vagina. When this exists, it may be
torn and bleed in the first union; but it is wanting in
so many cases, and may be distended or ruptured in
so many ways, that, though its presence is held to be
sufficient proof of virginity, its absence is not a certain
indication of the contrary.

The clitoris, placed above the opening of the urethra, is a miniature, imperfect penis, capable of erection, and, in the sexual congress, receiving, from the
friction of the parts where it is situated, the most vivid
excitement of pleasure. This excitement may also be
produced artificially, as in the male organ, but with
great loss of nervous power, and, if habitual, it destroys
the sensibility of the part, while it wrecks the health of
the whole system.

The bosom, containing the milk-forming glands of
the female, is closely connected with the generative

organs in function and sympathy, partaking of their excitements. The nipple, indeed, in structure and erectile power, closely resembles the penis and clitoris. I shall describe it more particularly in connection with the glandular system and the function of lactation.

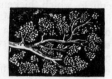

Fig. 21.—Mammary Glands.

The skin, or external covering of the body, is a vast network of areolar tissue, fibrous, elastic, and very strong—as we see it in leather, from the thickest sole-leather to the most deli

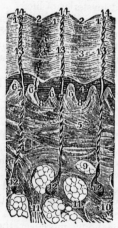

Fig. 22.—Magnified Section of the Skin of the Sole of the Foot. *

* 3, Epidermis; 4, Rete Mucosum; 5, Cutis Vera; 6, Papillæ; 9, Fat-cells; 12, Sweat Glands; 13, Sweat Canals; 14, Pores.

cate glove-leather—through which is spread a network of arteries, veins, lymphatics, nerves, and glands ; and it is protected on the surface by a horny scarf skin, or cuticle, which thickens into nails at the ends of the fingers and toes. Millions of pores allow the passage of perspiration, or waste matter of the body, through the skin. By its nerves we have the sense of feeling, of temperature, and the influences of air light, and electricity, and are affected with a variety of impressions. Over the whole body hairs grow from the skin, of matter similar to the cuticle, and performing some function of which little is known. Why the hair should be thick and long on certain parts and not on others, and why men have beards and women have not, are among the myriad mysteries of life.

The skin is continued into the alimentary canal, where it becomes a soft membrane, constantly lubricated by the mucous secreted from the blood by its glands, as perspiration, and an oily fluid softens the skin. Other membranes, very fine and shining, moistened with a more watery fluid, line the brain, lungs, and intestines. An excessive secretion, or lack of the power of re-absorbing this serous fluid, constitutes dropsy.

The joints are also provided with a membrane called the synovial membrane ; and its secretion, serum, with an unusual amount of albumen, like the white of an egg, lubricates every joint.

The eye is also constantly moistened with the secretion of the lachrymal gland, placed at the upper outer corner of the eye for that purpose.

All through the body, moreover, the arteries pour out a perspiration to keep the whole areolar tissue moist, and this is as constantly taken up by the veins. When the equilibrium of this process is disturbed, we have dryness and hardening of the tissues in one case, or œdema, or general dropsy in the other.

The average stature of men at birth is 1·64 feet (one foot and 64 hundredths); at 2 years, 2·60; at 4, 3·04; at 6, 3·44; at 9, 4·00; at 15, 5·07; at 20, 5·49; at 40, 5·52; after which age it slightly diminishes, from the curving of the spine and solidification of cartilages. Women at birth are 1 foot 61 hundredths; at 2 years, 2·56; at 4, 3·00; at 6, 3·38; at 9, 3·92; at 15, 4·92; at 20, 5·16; at 40, 5·18.

The average weight is, of men at birth, 7·06 pounds; at 15, 96·40; at 20, 132·46; at 40, 140·42.   That of women is, at birth, 6·42; at 15, 89·04; at 20, 115·30; at 40, 121·81.

Men and women at mature age weigh twenty times as much as at birth, and their stature is three and a quarter times greater.

A calcined human body weighs only 8 ounces; mere drying reduces it to one-tenth of its weight.   Thus nine-tenths of the whole body are water.

CHAPTER IV

PRINCIPLES OF PHYSIOLOGY.

THE primitive form of organic life is a cell, or vesicle. As seen under the microscope, there is a cell within the cell, or a nucleus, and within that a point called nucleolus—cell within cell.   It is in this manner that matter, under the influence of what we may call vital force, takes an organic form.   It has parts, an ext io pellicle or skin, and an interior, filled with fluid.

The cell is the beginning of every organised bein —from the simplest vegetable to the highest animal- in each case we have but a microscopic point.   It ma be developed into a toad-stool or an oak, a worm or philosopher; but at its beginning and in a certain stage of its progress it would be very difficult to tell one from the other. They have the same appearance under the microscope, and are composed of the same elements. But in the microscopic germ—in this simple watery cell—is the vital intelligent force that determines and accomplishes its development.

A cell may divide itself into two, and these into four, and so on; and by this kind of multiplication, there may be a rapid growth; or a cell, containing within itself several smaller cells, may burst, and each of these may, in turn, develop, generate, and dissolve. In one way or other the organic being increases and multiplies.

Under the moulding power of a force, guided by intelligence, which presides over the growth of each plant and animal—the soul and guiding power of the organism — these cells take on all organic forms. Flattening, the cells become membrane; elongating, they are fibres; joining together, by an absorption of their joining parts, they form tubes; and so of all the organised tissues. In this way we have woody fibre, sap tubes, and all the parts of the vegetable, from its first leaf to its flower and perfect fruit. In the same way, we have cells forming blood-vessels, muscle, nerves, and all the most complicated and beautiful organs of the human body.

But before a cell can be formed there must be matter suitable to its formation. We have here the principles necessary to form a universe. There must be matter and the intelligent forming spirit. This matter out of which cells are formed is called proto-plasm or blastema. It is essentially albuminous, and the egg of the common fowl, out of which is formed all the parts of the chicken, is the type of all blastema.

It is believed by some that the blastema may take on the forms of simple fibrous tissue and basement membrane, without passing through the cellular trans-

formation. These parts are less vital than others, and
less subject to decay, while the whole cellular substance of the system—all parts generated by cell
growth—is in a constant process of change, of dissolution and reproduction. Each of the myriad cells that
goes to make up the human body, seems to have its
own birth, life, and death; it dissolves, is carried away,
and another cell takes its place. All vital processes,
even those of thought, are accompanied by the destruction and reproduction of cells; and hence the
necessity for constant nutrition and constant excretion
—the perpetual supply of new materials, and the conveying away of the waste matter.

Thus it is in the human body, as in the human race.
The individual cell dies and another takes its place,
but the body lives on. The individual man dies, the
life of the race continues. In the human body we
have an elaboration of alimentary matter into blood,
and from this blood is formed the cells of all the vital
tissues. All analogy points to the birth, growth,
maturity, decline, and death of the human race; the
same as in the individual man. And it may be that
planets and systems are subject to the same law.
We appear to be in the early period of our planet
and our race. We look forward to the maturity and
happiness of both man and earth—man, of which each
individual forms a part—the earth, our home.

Let us love and beautify this home; let us try to
educate and benefit this humanity. No organ of the
body, no cell which adds its almost infinitesimal life to
the structure of an organ, can be isolated from the
other organs and cells. Complete in its individuality,
it is yet held in the bonds of closest sympathy. One
life pervades all—one spirit governs all. If one is
happy, all rejoice; if one is diseased, all suffer. So it
is with the individual man and the race. Each man
has his own individual life—his rights, his happiness—

but a bond of social sympathy and a great soul of
humanity pervades the race. All humanity suffers for
the disease or wickedness of any individual; all humanity is ennobled by every great deed. These are
mysteries; but life and death and immortality are
mysteries. The universe is a mystery; the fact of our
existence, and of the existence of our system, and
planet and race, are profound mysteries.

But they are mysteries that we shall solve. God
has not mocked His human children with wants never
to be satisfied, curiosity never to be gratified, and aspi-
rations never to be made realities. Nature is our
book, and we hold in our own organisation and consciousness the key of all mysteries.

In a certain sense, God may be said to be the soul
of the universe—its guiding, informing spirit; and every
organised being, whether vegetable, animal, or man, is
pervaded by a spiritual principle, which acts upon
matter, moulds it to its own form, and controls the
whole phenomena of organic life, consciousness, passion, and intelligence. We see everywhere in nature
the proofs of intelligent design, not merely working
outwardly, but inwardly, as the Apostle says, " God
working in us, both to will and to do."

It may not be readily admitted that the operations
of organic life are controlled by a pervading intelligence; but I see no way of escaping this conclusion.
When the tendril of a climbing plant reaches out to its
supporter; when the roots of a rose-tree travel directly
toward water, surmounting all obstacles, and changing
their course as the position of the water is changed;
when I see plants, growing in partial darkness, reaching toward a ray of light, upward, sideways, and even
downward, as the ray is changed; when I see the
flowers of two plants of opposite sexes inclining to
each other, and coming together to consummate their
nuptials, or the male organ of a flower, which is the

love-shrine of both sexes, bending downward or reaching upward to embrace its feminine partner; when I see the pistil, or female organ of a flower, surrounded by several loving stamens, bend first to one and then the other, to receive the vivifying influence from each, I see signs of intelligence. "But that intelligence," you say, "is external to the plant or flower; it does not reside in it." How do you prove that? Why not say, as well, that the intelligence of the ant, or bee, or canary bird, or dog, or elephant, are external, and do not belong to them?

And in the operations of the animal organisation, the merely vegetative functions, I see evidence of the same intelligent action. When we tie the large artery that supplies the leg with blood, the limb is first cold and numb; it calls for its accustomed supply of nutriment, but the channel is closed. What is done? Pretty soon a warmth is diffused through the limb. The small arteries below, that interlace with those above the ligature, enlarge themselves so as to supply the limb with blood. Here seems to be the consciousness of a want, and that want supplied by the most intelligent operations. Where does that intelligence reside? If you cut a hydra into twenty pieces, where is the intelligence that forms for each part all the other parts that belong to it, so as to make twenty perfect animals?

So, if a bone is broken, the nerves and vessels about the fracture set to work as intelligently as so many bees to mend their comb. They demand and receive a large supply of blood; they separate from it the materials of bone; first the gelatine, and then the earthy matter. They form a plug of bone in the hollow of the shaft, and then a ring of bone around it. Having made it temporarily secure, they then set to work, deposit and build up the bone where it should be, and finally remove the temporary plug and ring of

bone, leaving the part with scarcely any mark of fracture. Where is the intelligence that presides over this
complicated and beautiful operation? In the brain?
There is not the least evidence of it. The whole
process would go on just as well without a brain—
for the whole body of an infant has been perfectly
formed without brain.

These intelligent operations take place continually,
in every part of the body, from the beginning of its
development to the end of life. A thousand facts
prove that each organ, each cell, and each atom has
its own life, in harmony with, and contributing to the
general life, or the spirit which pervades the whole.
And when this material organisation shall have per
formed its uses, and is laid aside at death, the spirit
continues to exist, parted from the earthly envelop-
ment, but retaining force and form.

It would seem that matter is a temporary accident;
spirit a more permanent and higher reality. This
state of existence seems to be a necessary condition
of our spiritual progress. Our earthly life is a real
necessity, and a real blessing, and we should endeavour to improve and enjoy it in all its integrity
and force. We should give ourselves all the advantages of a full, healthy, integral life; a life of energy,
activity, beauty, and enjoyment. The standard of a
true life is its amount of happiness; and happiness
comes from the fullest and highest exercise of all the
passions of the human soul—from a life full of the
highest harmonies. We are not to despise this life,
its uses, and its enjoyments. God has given it to us
for a noble purpose, and it is our duty to enjoy what
He has given us. Our bodies, then, are worth understanding, and worth taking care of.

In considering the bodily life of man, we may class
his organs and functions into three groups, which may
be distinguished as the Vegetative or Organic, the

Sensitive or Animal, and the Generative. By the vegetative or organic system, I mean the functions and organs connected with nutrition—the building up, growth, and nourishment of all parts of the body. This system has its own nervous organisation, the sympathetic or ganglionic, with nervous centres governing digestion, the formation of blood, its circulation, absorption, secretion, &c.

The animal system consists of the organs and faculties of sensation, locomotion, thought, feeling, passion, and spirituality.

The generative function is connected with both systems of organs, and requires for its perfection the exercise of all the powers of both, in their highest development and vigour.

These three great functions are named here in the order of their development and action. The body is built up cell by cell, and organ by organ, from its primitive form, by the nerves of organic life acting upon the nutritive processes. The brain and senses are inactive in the fœtus; but the heart pulsates, the capillaries are at work, and the body is prepared for independent life. Under the intelligent agency of the nerves of organic life, all the structures of the body are perfected. We have that beautiful optical instrument, the eye, which our best artists can only bunglingly imitate, formed in the darkness of the womb. We have the complicated apparatus of hearing, still less understood, silently elaborated; and the still more astounding organ of thought. They are all formed ready for action; but they are all at rest, until, at the end of the nine months of gestation, independent life begins, and the animal powers are added to the organic. The child breathes, then it exercises the propensity of alimentiveness; and, day by day, it gradually acquires the power and use of its intellectual and moral faculties.

This striking difference is to be noticed between the organic and animal organs. The first require no education. They act perfectly from the beginning. The heart beats as well when it is a pulsating point beneath the microscope, as at any subsequent period. The capillaries and glands need no training to perform their offices. But the animal organs require exercise and education. It is true that those most intimately connected with organic life, act with an instinctive spontaneity; such as sucking, swallowing, etc.; but locomotion, language, and the exercise of the mechanical and intellectual powers, comes to the human being by slow degrees, and the higher faculties come one after another into their development and action.

Another difference is in relation to consciousness. If a man were not told, he would never know that he had heart, stomach, liver, kidneys, and any of the internal organs of nutrition. Even with all the aids of scientific observation, what ages elapsed before the circulation of the blood was discovered? From the time food is swallowed, until it enters into the structure of our organs, lives its brief organic life, dies, and is conveyed out of the system, we have no particular consciousness of any of the changes through which it passes. In health there is a general feeling of satisfaction and pleasure in the performance of every function; but this feeling is vague. In disease, these acts may be accompanied by pain.

But it is the law of the organic system, that its functions are unconscious and vaguely pleasurable in health—and that these nerves only acquire sensation in disease, when they produce pain by their connection with the nerves of sensation belonging to the nervous system of animal life.

A good digestion, a brisk circulation, a vigorous action of the capillaries and corresponding secretions, give a general feeling of health, and a degree of

pleasure of which we are hardly conscious, until, by
being deprived of it, we have data for comparison.
To have made us conscious of these incessant actions
of our vegetative life, might have been a discomfort.
While they all go on rightly, it is enough for us to
have the general and pleasant feeling that all is right;
but when there is food in the stomach that cannot be
digested, poisons in the system that cannot be elimi-
nated, nature cries out against the outrage, and her
warning cry is *Pain*.

The grand centre of the superadded functions of animal life is the brain. Here is the centre of consciousness,
of sensation, of voluntary motion, of thought, of passion.
The brain, and its appendages, the spinal cord, and the
nerves of sensation and motion, are built up and constantly nourished by the vegetative functions. The
perfection of human organisation is the proper proportion between the development and activity of these two
classes of functions, and of the third to these.

The brain is an organ of slow growth, and requiring
practice for the due exercise of its organs. This is
true of thought, as well as of voluntary motion. We
learn to reason as we learn to walk; we require practice in thinking as we do in dancing.

There is no power of the soul that may not be
developed and strengthened by exercise, or crushed
by repression, or weakened by inaction. But you cannot train the beatings of the heart, nor educate the
peristaltic motions of the bowels. All you can do for
the vegetative organs is to give them good conditions.
For the animal powers you may do much more. The
former may be perverted, weakened, and destroyed,
so also may the latter, but they may also be educated
to an unknown degree of power and perfection. In
health, the stomach, heart, and other organs of the
vegetative system will act alike in the most ignorant
savage and the greatest genius.

Everywhere the organic nerves mingle with those of animal life. The vigour of brain and muscle depend upon the perfection of nutrition, and the processes of nutrition are greatly influenced by our thoughts, feelings, and movements.

The third function, or system of functions, is still later in development and action. Neither the cerebellum, believed by phrenologists to be the seat of amativeness in the brain, nor the sexual organs, attain their full size and power of healthy action until the age of ten to eighteen years, varying with climate and constitution. But even at the age of puberty, the system is still too immature for the highest and most perfect exercise of the procreative power. Men and women should come to maturity before they can give the best mental and bodily constitutions to their posterity.

CHAPTER V.

OF THE ORGANIC SYSTEM.

IN the organic or vegetative system, we have to consider:—

1. The acting force, or element of vitality residing in the ganglionic nervous system. Of the nature of this life force we know nothing; and we can only observe its laws or mode of action.

2. The matter acted upon; and this is the blood, or nutritive fluid, from its formation by the assimilation and vitalisation of aliment, to the last and highest products of secretion and elimination.

3. The apparatus of various kinds by which these processes are performed, as the organs of digestion,

absorption, assimilation, circulation, respiration, nutrition, secretion, excretion.

The central thing here is the blood, and we have to consider the relation of the blood to the food from which it is formed; to the atmosphere by which it is purified and vitalised; and to the organs and functions of animal life.

This order, rendered as simple as possible, may still seem complicated, but in a system in which all the parts are so interwoven, and mutually dependent, no plan can wholly free us from complexity.

For example, if, in explaining the process by which blood is formed from food, I begin with the chewing of this food, and its being mixed with saliva, I stumble at the very outset upon a process of secretion. The blood makes saliva, and the saliva helps to make blood. The blood makes gastric juice, and the gastric juice helps to convert food into blood. This is the fact, also, even with regard to the active force which presides over these processes. The vital force, or ganglionic nervous power, assimilates nutritive matter, and vitalises it into the living fluid blood—but it is the blood that nourishes these nerves, and gives them vital force. The blood makes the nerves, and the nerves make the blood. So the blood builds up and nourishes the heart, arteries, and veins that carry it over the system. And we shall find that to a greater or less degree this reciprocity of influences extends to all the processes of life.

Considering the acting force, or nervous power, as only to be understood by its effects, let us now consider this reservoir of life, the blood, in its various functions and relations. It is a thin red liquid of a bright scarlet colour, when drawn from an artery; but of a deep crimson, or purple, when it comes from a vein, and venous and arterial blood differ as much in their properties and constituents. The quantity of blood in a healthy middle-sized man is estimated at 25 or 28 pounds, or about one-fifth the weight of the body.

When allowed to stand for some hours after being drawn, the blood separates itself into two portions, a central, solid portion, called the clot, and a yellow watery serum. The clot is composed of a mass of fibrin, which has drawn together, in its meshes, a quantity of blood discs, or flattened cells, about one five-thousandth of an inch in diameter, which contain the red colouring matter.

Blood consists of water, fibrin, albumen, and some mineral constituents. Its most important ultimate elements are carbon, hydrogen, oxygen, and nitrogen, and it contains the materials necessary for the nutrition of every tissue of the body, and the matter of all secretions. The milk, bile, urine, fœcal matter, perspiration, saliva, tears, are all in the blood, actually existing, or with their elements ready to be combined.

This blood is constantly circulating through the system. It passes through the heart at the rate of about five hundred pounds an hour. All this passes through the heart, and passes through the lungs, where, through a million tubes, it rushes in a full stream, like an ever-rushing river, coming in contact with the air we breathe. Then it all pours through the great aorta, branching out, like a vast tree, and it goes on until every atom of the body is supplied with the fresh, bright, arterial fluid.

Without it is no motion, no sensation, no life. Check for an instant the current of blood to the brain, and you have syncope; prevent its becoming arterialised by contact with oxygen, and you have the insensibility of asphyxia. It is not blood only, then, that is necessary to sensation and life, but oxygenated, arterial blood—blood of a certain chemical organisation.

This blood is alive. It is as much alive as any

muscle or nerve in the body. A dead liquid would not answer, in contact with living tissues. And this conversion of dead matter into living blood is one of the mysteries. It is life that begets life, and it is the vitality constantly generated in the nervous centres of the organic system, that gives life to the blood.

When blood is drawn, it does not die at once. Its clotting is a vital operation. If the blood is killed at once by a stroke of lightning, it never clots, but soon turns putrid. Some blood clots and turns putrid more slowly than other. Strong, healthy blood is longer in going through these processes than weak, sickly blood. The human blood that is made from pure vegetable food, will keep whole days longer than blood made by living on the flesh of other animals.

The assimilation of nutritious matter, the formation of the primitive blood globules, and their vitalisation, appear to take place in the lacteal and lymphatic glands, under the influence of the nerves of organic life. In this system we have matter brought from all parts of the body, passing through great numbers of these glands; we have also the matter absorbed from the intestines, by the process of cellular formation and dissolution; matter from each death rising to a higher life; and all this matter goes to mingle with the general current of the blood. In it may be seen, by the microscope, the lymph globules, white, clear, but destined to imbibe colouring matter, and become red globules.

But before we go farther, let us glance a moment at the structure and action of glands. All vital actions seem to be carried on by means of surfaces. The more important the operation, the greater the surface concerned. A simple membrane gives a certain extent of surface; we have still more in cells, and still more when these cells line tubes, and those tubes increase their length by multiplied convolutions.

In the human body we have all sorts of glandular apparatus, from a single follicle, or depression, up to the immense convolutions of the seminal tubes in the testicle, or the still more complicated nervous tubuli in the nervous centres.

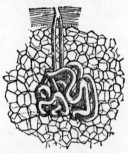

Fig. 24.—A Sweat Gland from the Palm of the Hand, magnified 40 diameters.

Wherever any vital action is to be performed, we have, by some means, an extent of surface proportional to its importance. In the lungs, the air-cell surface is estimated at 1500 square feet. In the same organ the convolutions of capillary vessels, in which the blood is brought to imbibe oxygen from the air and give off carbonic acid, must make a surface many times greater. The vessels and secreting cells of the liver contain a vast amount of surface. The kidneys are a compact mass of tubes. Through a vast net-work of mesenteric glands, the chyle passes, on its way to be converted into blood.

The lacteal and lymphatic glands, which are of a similar character, and which probably perform a similar office, are liable to be diseased, by poisonous matter passing through them. Thus in the absorption of syphilitic matter, large swellings, called buboes, are formed in the groin, where there is a mass of these glands. Similar buboes, but not of so malignant a character, sometimes arise from gonorrhœa. The glands of the neck are swollen in scrofula, and sometimes those in the armpits. But when the glands of the mesentery are diseased to any considerable extent, the result is a slow, wasting consumption. The system demands blood, the blood demands its aliment, the stomach feels the demand in a craving appetite, but the channels of communication are cut off. The glands cannot perform their function. The system wastes; its matter is used over and over to make new blood, as long as it will answer for this purpose; but this cannot go on. The patient sinks into a hopeless marasmus, and literally starves to death. This disease is called consumption of the bowels, to distinguish it from the consumption of the lungs.

There are going on in every part of the system the most constant and rapid processes of secretion, or the separation of various matters from the blood, and the additions to the blood must correspond with these, to keep up the equilibrium of life. After arriving at his full growth, a man may live on for many years, scarcely ever varying in weight. He consumes tons of food, and gives off tons of excretions. There may be a gradual deposition of fatty matter in the cells of the areolar tissue, a stock of food laid up for the wants of age, when the partial failure of digestion may render such a supply convenient; but this variation is but slight in ordinary cases. Day by day, consumption and waste very nearly balance each other.

The reader may have already perceived that there are two modes by which matters get into the blood, and they get out of it in a similar manner. One mode is by simple mechanical absorption or transudation; the other is a more vital process, and is performed by means of glands, or cells, under the influence of organic nerves. For example, if a pint of water is taken into the stomach, when demanded by thirst, it is sucked up by the veins as by a sponge. In a feverish state of the system, if a pint of water is injected into the rectum, it is also quickly absorbed into the circulation. The veins of the skin also absorb water in bathing, and even from the atmosphere.

Water is not digested, but is itself the great digestive agent. It undergoes no change, unless by analysis and synthesis, but is simply absorbed. This is also the fact respecting many substances dissolved in water, or themselves liquid; and this is the reason why water for drinking should be soft and pure. Alcohol passes from the stomach directly into the circulation as alcohol, by venous absorption. It passes through the liver, exciting and disordering that organ. It is carried by the blood to the brain, producing exhilaration, intoxication, and finally stupefaction. It passes off by the lungs, tainting the breath, by the skin, by the kidneys, and doing mischief everywhere. Pure alcohol can be distilled from the blood, brain, breath, or urine of the drunkard. If the finger be dipped in spirits of turpentine, in a few minutes it can be smelled in the urine. Many things get into the blood through the lungs. If we breathe the vapour of chloroform or ether for a few moments, it taints the breath for many hours, having been absorbed into the blood and gradually expelled again. Thus we may be poisoned in our food, our drink, in the air we breathe, and by the substances we come in contact with. And in each case it is the blood that suffers, and through the blood the nerves of both animal and organic life. And as the blood has its own life, the blood may be fatally poisoned, and this is unquestionably the fact in cer tain epidemic and contagious diseases.

But the most important and vital portions of the blood are received by means of another and a more elaborate kind of absorption, or assimilation. The small intestines are covered with villi, or minute excrescences, millions in number, and presenting a vast surface, having no openings, but containing an apparatus of blood-vessels and nerves, where, by a process of cell formations and dissolutions, the matter of nutrition is received into the circulation.

Before food can become chyle, and from chyle be vitalised into blood, it must be comminuted and dissolved---dissolved so thoroughly as to pass through

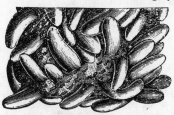

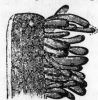

Fig. 25.— Villi and Follicles of Ileum, highly magnified.

Fig. 26.—Longitudina. Section of Small Intestines, showing Villi.

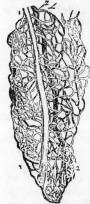

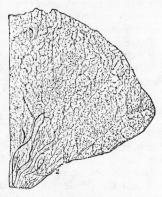

Fig. 27.—Arteries and Veins of an Intestinal Villus, magnified 45 diameters : arteries dark.

Fig. 28.—Injected Veins from Coat of Intestine.

animal membrane, like water or oxygen. And it does become so by the process of digestion. It is mashed, or should be, by the teeth; it is moistened and partly

dissolved by the saliva, which flows into the mouth
just when it is wanted, from three pairs of glands.   It
is lubricated by mucous glands around the roots of
the tongue, in the pharynx and esophagus.

Arrived in the stomach, with digestion well begun,
the blood gathers around this organ, and distends its
coats.   From this blood the gastric glands secrete the
gastric juice, with its basis of hydrochloric acid, and
its wonderful dissolving power.   It is poured from the
orifices of minute follicles, opening in the folds of the
mucous membrane.   Of these follicles there are two
hundred and twenty-five in the square of the eighth
of an inch; fourteen thousand four hundred in a
square inch, or one million two hundred and ninety-
six thousand follicles to the entire stomach, and each
of these follicles the outlet of a complex glandular
apparatus, surrounded by a dense net-work of blood-
vessels and nervous fibres.

These follicles, pouring out the secretions necessary
to the digestive process, or giving exit to matter which
is to be excreted from the bowels, extend through the
whole length of the alimentary canal.   In the five feet
length of the colon, these follicles are very close and
minute, and their number is estimated at nine millions
six hundred and twenty thousand.

But even this vast amount of surface—and all the
length, convolutions, and folds of the intestines are to
give surface; all these glands, follicles, and villi, are
surface—is not enough.   To pour a kind of salivary
fluid into the duodenum, or small intestine near the
stomach, we have a glandular mass called the pancreas,
weighing several ounces; while the liver is a mass of
glands separating bile from the blood, weighing four
or five pounds.

We get a much clearer idea of the organs of the
body, when we consider each individual portion—
each villosity, or each follicle, as a distinct organ,

performing its appropriate function. But however minute these may be, we must go further, and consider each cell as the final individual, in which resides the functional power. And each cell is formed by the nervous power, and performs its function under nervous influence. Withdraw the nervous power from the salivary glands, and the parched mouth receives no saliva. Under a sudden paralysis of the nervous system, from some shock, the tongue cleaves to the roof of the mouth, the food sticks in the unlubricated throat; no gastric juice is poured into the stomach, and the food, lying a dead weight, oppresses the organ, or irritating like any foreign substance, produces nausea and vomiting; the action of the bowels ceases, and we are affected by constipation, or in their relaxation, have diarrhœa. All this disorder comes from a disturbance of the nervous equilibrium.

When the food has been transformed into blood, its vitalisation is not completed until it has been brought in contact with the atmosphere. The blood is a living fluid, and, like all living beings, *it must breathe.* And it demands pure air. No sooner has it passed into the right side of the heart, than it is thrown into the lungs, where every drop gathers around a vesicle of air. It asks for air, with an importunity that will not be denied. We cannot withhold the supply. The blood must breathe. It must have oxygen. Each blood disk rushes to the net-work of fibres, which we call membrane, sends off its atom of carbonic acid, and receives its atom of oxygen, blushing like a bride. In the capillaries it finds tissues which want oxygen.

The action of the blood in the capillaries is obscure It turns from arterial to venous, changing its colour from scarlet to purple; loses oxygen, and receives carbonic acid. New matter is deposited in the tissues by cellular appropriation, and the waste matter is removed, and in this process there is an evolution of animal heat. All this takes place under the influence of the nerves of organic life. And, in every minutest part, this nervous power seems to exercise an adaptive intelligence, which provides, to a great extent, and as far as possible, for all exigencies.

And now the blood, having eaten its food, and breathed its air, and performed its work in the capillaries, where it builds up with new, and whence it conveys whatever rubbish of the old matter, must be relieved of its burden, and kept sweet, pure, and vigorous, that it may give sweetness, purity, and vigour to all parts of the system, and especially to the brain and special organs of the soul, to which it first and chiefly ministers.

For this purpose, we have a set of cleansing organs. Some of these have been already noticed. The fæcal matter is poured from the blood-vessels in the mucous membrane of the intestines, through millions of openings; and this action of the bowels is one of the conditions of health. The liver separates from the blood a great mass of carbonaceous matter, which, while assisting in digestion, is not the less excrementitious; and if the action of the liver ceases but for a day, the skin is tinged with the yellow hue of the retained bilious matter.

Two large branches of the abdominal aorta convey powerful currents of arterial blood to the kidneys, which, by a complicated and beautiful apparatus, separate from it the urine, full of the waste nitrogenised matter of the tissues. Here is muscular matter with its sulphur, and nerve matter with its phosphorus. Here is the ammonia, formed by the combination of nitrogen and hydrogen. Here are salts and minerals, the latter, when in excess, sometimes forming gravelly and stony accretions. The kidneys are vital organs; for, if the matters they separate from the blood, and send off to the bladder, through the ureters, were retained, they would poison the blood to putrefaction, and paralyse the brain to coma.

The skin is not less important as a great depurating organ. I call the skin an organ, as I do lungs, liver, kidney. Like them, it is a vast collection of individual organs; each at work by itself in this great process of purification. Like the lungs and alimentary canal, the skin has internal functions, as well as external. The blood breathes by the skin, receives oxygen; and it is through this avenue

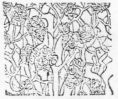

Fig. 29.—A Portion of Kidney magnified 60 diameters.

that it gets the life-giving influence of light, and aromal influences, electrical, magnetic or mesmeric, and miasmatic. The skin, even with its covering of horny cuticle, offers but little impediment to such liquids as water, alcohol, spirits of turpentine, etc., and the gases travel through it without hindrance.

Franklin's air-bath was a very common-sense discovery of a *very* common-sense philosopher. We may be invigorated or poisoned through the skin. It is a truly vital organ. Let a certain portion of its surface be destroyed by any means, and death is inevitable. The Frenchman who covered a little boy with gold-leaf, to make him look like a California cupid, killed him as surely as if he had put a ligature around his windpipe. The water-cure physicians have by no means over-rated the importance of the skin.

Like the mucous membrane of the intestines, the skin is everywhere pierced with follicles, here called pores, each of which is the outlet of a gland, formed by the convolutions of the tube, and around which is a mesh of blood-vessels and nerves. These glands perpetually separate from the blood, and these exc

F

tory ducts pour out, the matter of perspiration. This passes off in vapour, unless it is in such a quantity that the atmosphere cannot take it up fast enough, when it gathers in liquid drops of sweat.

The matter of this secretion varies with the state of the constitution, and the condition of this and other organs, which are engaged in the same general work of purification. When the circulation is active, and the skin healthy, every sudoriferous gland pours out the matter of perspiration. In violent exercise the whole skin is covered with it, and the garments saturated. Wherever there is an active determination to the surface we have this result. But, in this case, as in so many others, one act has several uses. The elimination of perspiration is a cooling process, as well as a purifying. When we increase the warmth of the body by any means, nature calls for the cooling process, and this call of nature is answered by a rush of blood to the glands of the skin, and the pouring out of this vapour, and the system is cooled by this process—so that men can bear the hottest climates, the Turkish bath, furnaces, and even ovens hot enough to bake food. In the blanket pack we determine to the skin by the accumulation of vital heat.

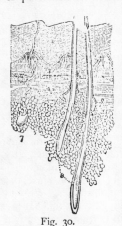

Fig. 30.
Vertical Section of the Skin magnified.

When the pores of the skin are closed by the constriction of cold, or the action of its glands is diminished by a weakened or diseased constitution, the work of the skin is thrown upon other organs.

The kidneys pour out more urine, the liver secretes more bile, the lungs are filled with exudations; sometimes the action of the bowels is heightened to a diarrhœa. Colds and catarrhs are the ordinary result of checking the perspiration, or "taking cold."

On the other hand, the skin is often compelled to perform the function of some internal organ. In torpid states of the liver, the skin is filled with bile. In disease of the kidneys, the perspiration has sometimes the distinct odour of urine; in obstinate constipation of the bowels, it has the smell of fæcal matter. In the same way, each of the secreting organs may act vicariously for some other.

Thus much here of the relations of the blood to its means of purification. We shall need all this when we pass from physiology to its application in hygiene, pathology, and therapeutics.

The evolution of animal heat seems, at the first glance, to be as simply a matter of chemistry as the warming of a house by the combustion of coal in a furnace. But is it really so? True, our food contains carbon and hydrogen. We take in at every breath a portion of oxygen. The oxygen combines with the carbon to produce carbonic acid, and with the hydrogen to produce water. This is a real combustion, going on all over the body, and heat is the necessary product of combustion. The chemists have weighed all these elements, and their products, and there can be no mistake about the facts; but there is still an element to be taken into the account—the element of nervous power or vitality. That controls the circulation of the blood, congesting it in the viscera of the chest and abdomen, or throwing it to the surface. That fills the capillaries, or empties them. That causes a limb to become pale and cold, or gives it the swelling, redness, and heat of a violent inflammation.

And though the organic bases the animal, the animal presides over the organic. The passions and emotions of the mind influence the most purely organic functions. The ardour of hope, or desire, may give warmth to the whole system, while disappointment or fear may chill the frame, and set the teeth to chattering. The emotion of jealousy may make the hands, in a few moments, turn deathly cold; or a happy love may make them glow with the fires of passion. A thought sends the hot blood to the face in blushes. Disappointed love gives the sensation of a hard, dull, aching oppression round the heart. The lungs are constricted, and relieve themselves by frequent sighs. The heart may even break from the excess of this passion, in its painful and discordant action. Many such facts will suggest themselves to the observing reader.

The manner in which demand governs supply in the organic system, is a proof that this law of supply and demand is fundamental, and therefore universal. In the water-cure, we practice constantly upon this principle. If we want blood and action in a part grown weak and diseased, we apply cold. The increased and urgent demand brings the supply; and, as power increases by exercise, there soon comes the habit of action, and a cure. Heat, in the whole system, as in its parts, is generated as it is required. Supply is in proportion to demand. Send a man to discover the North Pole, and he comes to not only endure, but to be quite comfortable, with the thermometer at 30 or 40 degrees below zero. Send him to the tropics, and he keeps cool by a copious perspiration at 100 degrees above. He can even sit in an oven heated to 300 degrees, while a potato is baking beside him. This power of adaptiveness belongs to the nervous system.

There is a set of organs belonging to the organic

system, termed the ciliary bodies, from their resemblance to the eyelashes. Of microscopic minuteness, they grow upon the epithelial cells, which pave the mucous membrane. They are found in the air-passages of the lungs and nostrils, in the fallopian tubes, vagina, and urethra, and the ducts of the glands, and in all animals down to the lowest species.

Standing upon these minute cells, these ciliary bodies, by millions, move continually, and with a rapidity that makes them invisible, until they become gradually slower with the death of the part. They have no perceptible connection with muscle, blood-vessel, or nerve. In animalcules, they are the source of rapid motions. In zoophytes, they surround the mouth, and force currents of water through the passages, for purposes of nutrition or respiration. Constant and powerful liquid currents may be seen whenever these animals are examined under the microscope. In the higher animals, they line the internal passages, and the effect of their action is to carry the fluids in their proper direction. They free the bronchial tubes, keep up the motion of the secretions, and propel the ova through the fallopian tubes to the uterus. What is very wonderful is, that if a very small piece of mucous membrane is cut off, removed entirely from the body, and placed under the microscope, this action will go on for hours. This, however, is no more remarkable, perhaps, than the powerful independent action of the heart in some of the lower animals. If the heart of a frog is removed from its body, and laid upon a table, it will continue to beat for some time; and it is said that the heart of a sturgeon (a large fish), hung up in the sun, has continued to beat until it creaked with dryness.

CHAPTER VI.

THE ANIMAL SYSTEM.

THE functions of animal life are—

1. Sensation, through the means of sight, hearing, smell, taste, and touch, or feeling; with a deeper sense transcending these, but seldom or partially developed, and vaguely known as impressibility; organs, the nerves of sensation.

2. Perception, intelligence, memory, passion, will; all those varied powers of mind or soul whose special organ is the brain.

3. Voluntary motion, including all language, natural and acquired, and all modes of expression; nerves of motion and the muscular system, with its relations.

The organism of this series is symmetrical, or made up of two halves. This is true of the bones, muscles, etc., of the motive system, of the senses, and of the brain and its nerves. In this respect, these organs differ notably from the heart, stomach, liver, the whole digestive apparatus, and the nervous system of organic life.

The brain is the organ of the mind; and in this expression we recognise the existence of a soul or spirit which thinks, feels, wills, and acts, of which the brain is the material instrument through which it acts upon nerves and muscles.

The best analysis and classification of the faculties and passions of man we have, has been made by the phrenologists, though still imperfect; for we are conscious of possessing faculties for which they have not discovered organs. And the division of the cerebral organs into those of propensities, sentiments, and intellectual faculties, is not quite satisfactory; for every power of the intellect, even Form, Order, or Number, may become a passion; while the sentiments and propensities seem to have the properties of intelligence. Conscientiousness and Benevolence do not seem mere blind impulses, and thought and memory are joined to feeling. The "intuitions of the heart" seem to be the rapid and powerful action of the intelligence that resides in every passion of the soul. Each faculty seems to be a combination of desire and intelligence, with powers of foresight and memory. The reflective powers, Comparison and Casuality, by which we discover the harmonies of relation and sequence, and the general "fitness of things," are the calm judges that must give final decision; but what is called the instinctive knowledge of right may be the intelligence of Conscientiousness. So Constructiveness, or what is called the propensity to build or construct, seems to carry with it in insects, birds, and higher animals, as well as in man, certain powers of intelligence and action; and I can conceive of no passion which is not accompanied by a kind of intelligence suited to its nature and objects, giving us the knowledge called instinctive or intuitive, and which, though liable to many perversions, is, in a true life, perhaps more reliable than the action of the so-called intellectual powers.

How a mass of grey and white matter, 95 per cent. water, made up of cells and tubes, a pulpy, almost liquid substance, in which it is difficult to trace organisation, can be the organ of feeling and thought, and the wonderful powers of perception, memory, and imagination, is quite inconceivable. The action of muscles and bones in locomotion is mechanical and obvious enough—but how the impulse to move, and the skill to write, or play on a musical instrument, acts in the soft matter of the brain, and is sent down the nerves, we can have no conception.

There appears to be an element which some have imagined to be electricity, or an analagous substance or force, which connects what we call spirit with what we call matter. There appears to be a nervous aura pervading and surrounding the body; passing off by voluntary action in what is called magnetising, or mesmerising, in the fascination of serpents, and not less in men and women who have the power of charming; and which may be the medium of supersensual powers which we call psychometric, intuitive, gifts of second sight, prophecy, and gifts of healing.

That what we call spirit can act on what we call matter, we have proof in every organised being. There is no greater miracle in this way than ourselves, when, for example, a thought or memory moves our muscles, or causes a secretion of tears; but we have now a vast accumulation of facts, which prove that the spirits which have become entirely independent of material organisation, can, under certain conditions, act upon not only living souls, but upon dead matter.

There are many thousands of persons of unimpeachable character for intelligence and veracity, who are witnesses of this class of phenomena. Raps are made of various intensity, from a slight and almost imperceptible crackling sound, to loud sonorous vibrations, which can be heard over the house, and produce a sensible jar around them. When questioned, these raps answer with an intelligence which shows that they are produced by invisible beings. Sometimes the physical demonstrations are of a very powerful character. Heavy tables are raised from the floor, or tilted from side to side, without disturbing the objects upon them. Musical instruments are played upon without visible hands. Persons are raised bodily from the floor, and carried through the air, contrary to all received notions of the laws of gravitation. Often the messages from friends who have passed from this state of existence, give the most striking proofs of identity; but whether such proofs are ever beyond question or not, there is abundant evidence of the existence and action of invisible intelligences.

There seems to be no reason for disputing the facts. I have not stated one to which I could not summon hundreds of witnesses, the oaths of any two of whom would send a man to the gallows. The theories invented to explain the phenomena upon other hypotheses than the existence of spirits, are very unsatisfactory. The simplest way is to accept the explanation of those who avow that they are the real agents in producing these effects. All the other explanations yet attempted are absurd. I can readily believe that there is much delusion connected with pretended spiritual agencies; and I see no reason to believe that spirits are more infallible out of the body than in it. Admitting these facts, we have proof of two things—of spiritual existence, independent of our present material organisation; and of the power of spirit to act upon even the gross forms of matter, through certain media, or with the presence of certain aromal conditions.

In our present organisation, the soul appears to act both independently and through the finer matter of the brain and nervous fluid, upon the bodily organs. Each faculty and passion of the soul has its own special organ, over which it presides as a soul; and as with the organs of the body, the individuality of these organs is consistent with perfect harmony, and their harmony produces individuality.

While the cellular surface of the brain seems to be the seat of the soul, its internal portion is made up of connecting fibres. The base of the brain appears to be the seat of sensation, where all external impressions are received. Here centre the nerves of sight, hearing, taste, smell, and the wide and varied sense of feeling. These sensations, it is supposed, are conveyed to their appropriate cerebral organs, where they become perceptions, and the food of thought, sentiment, and passion. The rays of light, passing through the crystalline lens of the eye, form a perfect camera obscura picture upon the retina; and the optic nerve conveys the idea of that picture to the mind. The perception *may* take place in the retina itself; for the nerve may as well convey a perception as the impression of which that perception is made. Vibrations of the atmosphere, striking upon the drum of the ear, produce impressions upon the complicated apparatus of hearing of all appreciable varieties of sound. The powers of these instruments are truly wonderful. The eye seems more simple than the ear, and we come nearer to understanding its beautiful mechanism; but the result is, in both cases, a mystery.

The senses of smell and taste seem to be very simple modifications of the great sense of touch. Atoms of matter come in contact with the olfactory nerve, and we have the delights of smell. Savours, mingling with the moistening saliva of the mouth, come in contact with the nerves in the papillæ of the tongue, and we experience the pleasures of taste. These are two sentinels set to guard the avenue to the stomach; and to see that no impure thing finds entrance to the sanctuaries of organic life; for as the organic nature supplies strength to the animal, it is the duty of the animal to watch over and protect the organic.

The sense of feeling pervades the whole body, and even the organs of the other senses. We cannot only taste with the tongue, but we receive by it sensations of form, size, roughness or smoothness, heat or cold. So the nose can itch, or smart, or tingle, as well as distinguish odours. The surface of the eye is the seat of the most acute sensibility. We feel everywhere with the nerves of the skin, but especially with the ends of our fingers. This sense has relation to many faculties and passions. Things feel hot or cold, dry or moist, smooth or rough, slippery or the reverse, sharp or dull, hard or soft, rigid or pliable, regular or irregular, circular or angular. In some organs a modification of the sense of feeling gives exquisite pleasure.

"There is a natural body, and there is a spiritual body." If an informing soul builds up, animates, makes use of this body, with all its organs and senses, then the spirit, or spiritual body, must consist of the soul or *sub-stance* of the natural body as a whole, and also in every minutest part. If we have a spiritual head, we must also have spiritual hands and feet. We must have spiritual eyes, ears, noses, mouths, tongues, teeth. And, if these, we must have spiritual brains and nerves; spiritual blood, heart, arteries, lymphatics; spiritual lungs, liver, kidneys, bladder; spiritual food, secretions, and excretions. I consider this existence of man, future and immortal, a proven fact; and if he exist, it must be in some form, and with some organisation. He exists as a living, thinking, acting, enjoying being. And our only possible conception of him is as the same identical spiritual being that we now see him, only that the material organisation, or the natural body, seems to be the necessary condition of a certain stage of spiritual life, and when that stage is passed, it is no longer needed. An early death is, therefore, a great misfortune, though it may often save one from greater evils; and life may be too long when the soul is imprisoned in an organisation no longer fit to perform its functions. How affecting, and yet how natural, are sometimes the longings of the aged to be set free from what they feel to be clogs of mortality! The dread of death in the young, and

the longing for death in the very aged, are equally
natural.

The soul finds its normal expression, in this stage
of life, by means of the nerves of motion and their
organs, the muscles. By their means the soul walks
about, runs, climbs, gathers food, builds dwellings,
gathers and creates objects of use and beauty, which
constitute material riches. By their means the soul
laughs in her hilarity, exults in her joy, glories in her
triumphs, or weeps over her misfortunes. And every
passion and faculty of the soul finds expression in this
outward action, the force of which is conveyed by
nerves, and acts upon the muscles of animal life.
They also, as we shall show, have a powerful influence over the organic system.

Thus the faculty of tune finds expression, through
nerves and muscles, in the production of vibrations of
air, as it passes through the larynx—the most simple,
and, at the same time, the most perfect of all musical
instruments. Guided by the sense of hearing, and
aided by other intellectual faculties, this passion for
music also finds its expression by means of various
instruments; and the art of music produced by so
complicated an organism, becomes itself an expression of many other passions.

So all faculties, all feelings, all passions of the soul,
find their natural expression, or natural language, in
movements, gestures, signs, language, all of which are
accomplished by the nerves of motion, originating in
the nervous centres, and imparting their stimulus, or
motive force, to the muscular system.

If I read to myself, there is sensation, perception,
and thought—perhaps emotion or passion. But if I
read aloud, there is added to these a complicated process of nervous action and muscular motion. Some
of the best examples of these combinations of mental
and physical action, may be found in the earnest

orator, or the impassioned actor, whose whole being is controlled by the direct influence of the passions he has the power of calling into temporary action; the great singer, who overcomes the most astounding difficulties of vocalisation, and impresses us with all the emotions the composer intended to convey; the accomplished violinist or pianist, who effects the same with his fingers upon an artificial instrument; the artist, who flings the expression of beauty and passion upon the canvas, and fastens it there for centuries.

The apparatus by which these effects are produced is complicated and obscure, both in its structure and its action. The nerves of motion which govern the movements of the muscles of the face, eyes, tongue, etc., pass through several openings in the base of the cranium; but they have their origin in the upper part of the spinal cord, or medulla oblongata; and are connected with all parts of the cerebrum and cerebellum. The nerves of motion, that supply the trunk and extremities, are given off in pairs from the spinal cord, and seem to have in that continuation of the brain nervous centres which supply them with the power of action, though their movements are usually under the control of the will. This, however, is not always the case. There are involuntary actions, both constant and occasional, which seem to centre in the grey matter of the spinal cord. Respiration, performed both by the muscles of the chest, and the diaphragm and abdominal muscles, goes on from the beginning to the end of life. It may be controlled by the will, but does not depend upon it. The sphincters of the bladder and rectum are also in constant action. The muscles of the pharynx, employed in swallowing, act the moment any substance passes the fauces. So of the acts of coughing, sneezing, and, to some extent, that of laughing. Many of these acts are performed when the brain is quiet in sleep, or in a state of coma, or apoplectic insensibility. The spinal cord is the brain of the body; and it is questionable whether all voluntary actions are not of a secondary character, prompted by the brain, and then executed by the spinal cord.

Many physiologists believe that one of the functions of the cerebellum is to combine and harmonise muscular motion. There is little doubt that the organs of the brain form a perfect society, arranged in series and groups, acting together, in a normal state, in perfect harmony, and carrying out their impulses by the best possible adaptations of organism. A central, combining, regulating, and harmonising power may well reside in the cerebellum, which is an organ of the most beautiful and complex character, and a source and reservoir of power and energy.

According to our use of the word soul, it may be applied to every being that is gifted with sensation, thought, passion, and volition. It is the spiritual principle of animal or sensitive life; and there is also a lower soul or animating principle of organic life, which belongs both to vegetables and animals. The brains of animals, far down the scale of being, are like those of man. There is the same kind of grey, cellular matter, and white fibrous; nerves of sensation and motion; organs of sense, and organs of motion; an animal system super-imposed upon the organic.

The higher animals have the same senses as man, some in greater, some in a lesser degree of perfection. The sensations, of which these are the instruments, intellectual perceptions, moral feelings, passions, and propensities, seem to differ very little from our own. Animals have also their own varied modes of expressive action, which, in many cases, are similar to ours. The dog has many of the intellectual faculties of man; his sensations are acute, and he does not lack in expression. He has memory, and often shows a good judgment or power of adapting himself to circumstances. He is proud, vain, benevolent to men, and to his own species, faithful to trusts, firm in his friendships, very affectionate, cheerful, playful, courageous. He even appears to possess a remarkable degree of impressibility and foresight. He has a perception of things invisible to us, and of approaching dangers. He dreams. He very evidently understands our words, and seems often to divine our thoughts.

These are psychical powers. In man, we call them spiritual—what shall we call them in the brute? Insects, birds, and the mammalia exhibit similar faculties of mind or soul. The elephant is, in his moral and intellectual character, perhaps even superior to the dog; and he owes less to the companionship of man. In clearness of apprehension, calm judgment, tenacity of memory, benevolence, and affection, and many valuable qualities of mind and heart, he compares favourably with many of our own species.

What can we infer respecting the soul, or spiritual principle that presides over the material organism of the dog or elephant? If we admit, as has been sometimes urged, that soul is indestructible, and therefore immortal, we must give these animals immortality. If an existing individuality can never be destroyed, what becomes of individualities of so striking a character? It is important that we understand our true relations to the animals; and it is a grave question how far we have a right to enslave, mutilate, torture, murder, and devour them.

NOTE.—In speaking of the intellectual and moral faculties of animals, I have used the words in their common or phrenological, rather than their philosophical or theological, meaning. There are evident however inexplicable, differences between the mind and soul of man and the faculties of the highest of the brute creation.

CHAPTER VII.

THE FUNCTION OF GENERATION.

THE generative function has for its special use the continuation of the species; and it is intimately connected with the highest processes of both the systems of organic and animal life. There is no action of the body, and no power of the soul, which does not enter into the complicated and beautiful process by which humanity exists, and new beings are created. For the performance of this great function, we have a peculiar power or passion of the soul; special organs in the brain; nerves of exquisite sensation; voluntary and involuntary nerves of motion, with their muscular apparatus; and the most complex organs of innervation, circulation, nutrition, and secretion, connected with the system of organic life. Through all her works, nature has taken peculiar care of this function, often raised it above all others, and sacrificed all individual interests to the general welfare.

To do justice to a subject of so much scientific interest, and having such important relations to the health and happiness of man, I must treat it with entire freedom. I write for those, and those only, who are ready to accept the truth, and who desire to live it. I must also give more space to its consideration, than to topics which may be found elsewhere satisfactorily elucidated.

In the inorganic world, there is deposition, accretion, aggregation, but no such thing as generation. Minerals do not produce after their kind. But the moment we pass the line which divides inorganic from organic nature — the moment we come upon the domain of life we have processes of reproduction,

The simplest vegetable cell, at a certain period of its growth, divides itself into two similar cells. Other cells produce smaller cells within their walls, and then, at maturity, dissolve, and set the young cells free. A little further on, and in more complex organisms, we have what is called the gemmiparous reproduction. A bud, separating from the parent stock, becomes an independent plant. This last process is found pretty high in the scale of vegetable life, and is often coincident with higher forms of generation. In propagating many plants we may either use a slip, or a tuber, or the seed. The lower orders of animals propagate their species in the same way as the lower forms of vegetables. In animalculæ, we have divisions and gemmations, or the throwing off of buds, as in vegetables.

We now come, in both the vegetable and animal world, to more complex organisation, and higher methods of propagation, and find two principles uniting to form a living embryo. In the vegetable world, nature has surrounded the generative function and the sexual apparatus with the most attractive qualities. In some animals, and in most plants, the process is performed by the male and female organs in the same individual; but in some plants, and all the higher animals, we have the two sets of organs necessary to the result in two bodies, male and female.

In all cases, in this mode of generation, we nave this simple fact. There must be formed an ovum, or egg, which is, in its essential part, a cell of microscopic minuteness; and at a certain stage of its evolution, this egg must be fecundated by the addition of the male principle. The masculine and feminine elements unite to form the perfect germ of a new being.

It is remarkable, that the parts of plants devoted to

G

the sexual function, are those we most prize for their beauty and fragrance. It is the flower of the plant which contains the generative organs. The centre of the flower—the home of beauty, and fragrance, and sweetness—is the nuptial couch, the bower of love, sacred to the mysteries of vegetable procreation. In the centre of this bridal chamber is the pistil, or female organ; its tube corresponds to the vagina, and below it is the ovary, where the egg is formed and fecundated. This is done by one or more stamens which surround the pistil, and which have the power of secreting the spermatic fluid, which, in the form of pollen, falls upon the stigma of the pistil. The stamen corresponds to the generative organs of the higher male animals. In some plants, as the Indian corn, the sexual organs are further apart. The male, or sperm-preparing organs, are at the top of the stalk, while the female organs are midway. The pollen from the "tassel" must fall upon the "silk," or there will be no corn. In other cases, the male and female organs are on different plants of the same species, and the pollen from the male plant is brought by winds or insects to the female flowers.

In like manner, there are animals which contain in themselves both male and female organs. In some, the ovaries and testicles are near each other, and they have the power of self-fecundation. In others, each individual performs the part of both male and female to some other of its species.

But in the higher animals, and in man, there is no such hermaphrodism. The sexes are distinct, and the possession of one or the other set of organs, and the capacity of performing one or the other of these processes of the generative function, make the striking differences between the two sexes.

In my brief sketch of anatomy, I have described, with some minuteness, the more obvious and external

features of the two sets of generative organs.   I
have now to give a more thorough and physiological
account of this function and its relations.   It divides
itself naturally into three parts:

1. The passional, or that connected with the soul,
and having its nervous centre in the cerebellum—the
amativeness of the phrenologists;

2. The sensational or active, connected with manifestations and the sexual congress;

3. The organic, or the evolution of germs and
spermatozoa, in the ovaries and testicles, and the
progressive evolution and final expulsion of the fœtus.

The order in which we treat of the three divisions
of this subject may not be very important; but, after
what I have said of the nature of the organic process
in plants and the lower animals, I prefer now to begin
with the higher passional sphere, and descend through
manifestations and results; though, as will be seen, in
this, as in all the other functions of man, these are
intermingled and reciprocally act on each other.

The passion of love in our earlier years has what
may be called a rudimentary development.   In very
young children we perceive signs of the sexual instinct.
It is naturally shown in a gallant fondness which little
boys have for their mothers, their older sisters, and
generally for the female sex.   At the same time, little
girls have a peculiar tenderness for their fathers and
male friends.

The cerebellum, which Dr. Gall has proved, by many
observations, to be the seat of this passion, is usually
small and immature in childhood, corresponding to
the state of the feeling, and of its special organs; and
it is not until the age of puberty that all the organs
are developed together.   But as there is a rudimental
activity in the passional sphere, there is also, in
many cases, some excitement in the organic.   The
boy, before he reaches his teens, has his imagination

excited with ideas of sexual pleasure; and his immature organs partake of this excitement. If, at this
time, he is so unfortunate as to find the means of
gratifying his propensity, he runs the risk of forever
disordering, or even destroying his virile powers, and
of wrecking his whole mental and bodily constitution.
With the young girl, the danger is equally imminent.
Her passions are as strong, and her power of gratification even greater. If, in maturity, some women
seem to have the capacity for greater and more frequent enjoyment than men, in childhood a far greater
number destroy all desire, and all power of enjoyment.

There are some children, born of parents with disordered amativeness, who inherit passional activities,
and organic excitabilities, which hurry them to swift
destruction. Mere infants, both male and female, fall
by a perverted instinct into habits of masturbation.
This is not simply a vice; it is a disease. I do not
say that all vices are not of the nature of disease;
but this early propensity to the use, and consequent
destruction, of the sexual organs, is a special disease
which demands earnest sympathy and prompt attention for its cure.

In a normal condition, there is considerable excitement of the reproductive system on the approach of
puberty. This period comes, in boys, at the age of
fifteen to seventeen; in girls, from thirteen to fifteen;
and later or earlier in exceptional cases. Boys and
girls, as they approach this age, are full of romantic
sentiment, which expresses itself in profound sighs, in
a sweet melancholy, a love of solitude, and in ideali-
sations of adored, rather than beloved objects.

It would seem, from the experience of many persons,
that the most natural love of a youth of fifteen, is a
mature woman of twenty-five or thirty; and that the
affections of a girl of a corresponding age, are most
likely to be bestowed upon some mature man. At a

later period, men love women of their own ages, and still later, they respond to the affections of those who are much younger than themselves. Such loves, at this period, are the most suitable that can be formed, and the least dangerous. Youthful ardour and impetuosity are tempered and guided by the wisdom of experience; but where two very young persons are thrown together, their passions are liable to burn out themselves, and leave but cinders of their possessors.

The first love of either man or woman, eternal as it may seem to them, is not usually lasting; and if an effort is made to compel it to constancy by the bonds of marriage, it often proves a disastrous experiment. Left to itself, the illusion vanishes, or the love settles into a calm and beautiful friendship.

When the period of puberty has fully arrived, there comes a wonderful change over the whole being. No after change, till death itself comes, is so rapid and important. Soul and body expand with new powers and new feelings. The boy finds a beard sprouting on his chin, and hair also springing on the pubes. His neck increases in size by the expansion of the cerebellum behind, and the larynx in front. With the expansion of the larynx, his voice sinks a full octave in its pitch. The organs of generation increase in size and excitability; and with idleness and luxury, there come voluptuous thoughts by day and dreams by night, with extreme danger of solitary or social gratification of the sexual instinct, which may be a cause of disease, impotence, epilepsy, insanity; and, in any case, of life-long regrets. The remedy is to know and guard against the danger, and to keep a perpetual activity of body and mind, with great temperance in food and drink. If all the forces of life are used in bodily exercise and mental culture, the great dangers of youth may be escaped.

Puberty, in the girl, brings no less remarkable

changes. There is no beard upon the face, but hair begins to cover the mons veneris. The larynx does not expand, nor the voice deepen, but the cerebellum, though always smaller than in the male, increases in size, and the body expands into the full mould of womanly beauty. The pelvis enlarges, giving breadth to the hips, and a graceful swing to the carriage. The mammary glands enlarge, producing in all healthily developed girls the beautiful bosom which sculptors and painters are never tired of showing us, which fashion exposes and modesty conceals. But the most striking change that takes place when the girl becomes a woman, is the commencement of a monthly discharge from the uterus, through the vagina, coincident with and dependent upon the ripening of the germs in the ovaries, and their periodical expulsion.

Both sexes are now apparently fitted for the performance of the sexual function. In the male, the testicles have secreted the spermatic fluid, and elaborated its vital part, the living spermatozoa; the seminal vesicles are filled with this fluid, ready to be discharged. In the female, the ovaries have begun to bring forth the ova, which contain the germs, which only require the presence of the spermatic fluid to be developed into human beings.

What now is the order of nature at this period? Her work, in the reproductive function, is begun, and goes on, month after month, in the female, and continually in the male. Every month, one or more eggs are thrown off from the ovary, pass down the fallopian tube, lodge in the uterus, and if not fecundated, perish, and are expelled as abortions. At the same time nature is forming, in the testicles of the male, millions of spermatic animalcules, any one of which might effect the fecundation of the extruded ovum.

Before we mourn over this sad seeming waste of

the elements of life, let us send through nature a glance of inquiry. How large a proportion of the early blossoms on our fruit trees never ripens into fruit! How many millions of the seeds of plants become the food of animals, and never carry out their design of reproduction! Of the millions of eggs which come from a single fish, how few ever produce young! Why should there be millions of spermatozoa in a single discharge of the spermatic fluid, when it is probable that only one can ever act upon the same ovum?

Nature is bountiful. Nature is prolific. Especially in relation to this function, nature has everywhere dealt with a liberal hand. Puberty in woman begins at fifteen, and the monthly evolution of ova continues till fifty, when the function ceases. If she has but a single egg each month, she produces four hundred and twenty. But many women throw off two, and even three, four, or five at a monthly period. Twins are not unfrequent, and in rare cases three, four, or more children are born at once. Thus, a woman who lives in single blessedness, may have produced and wasted the germs of a thousand human beings. But it is evident that most of this seeming waste is quite orderly and intentional. When a germ is fecundated, or impregnated by the presence of the masculine secretion, the production of germs is suspended during the nine months of pregnancy, and usually also during the whole period of nursing. A perfectly healthy woman, living in natural conditions, will thus have a child once in two years during the period of child bearing.

The activity of the generative organs in both sexes, the constant production of the spermatic fluid in males after the age of puberty, and the periodical production of germs by the female, has made some ignorant people imagine that there should be a corresponding exercise of the sexual organs—that the union of the sexes should begin at puberty, and continue through life; but this is an evident absurdity. For several years after puberty, neither the male nor the female has arrived at sufficient maturity to produce healthy offspring. During gestation and lactation—pregnancy and nursing—all physiologists are agreed that sexual union is unnatural, and injurious to mother and child. Finally, the capacity for producing germs, and consequent child-bearing, ceases in women at the age of forty-five to fifty-five, while men have the procreative powers to a much later period.

It is evident that the early activity of the generative organism is intended for the perfection of the individual, and not for the continuation of the species. Love ripens and expands the soul, and its organic elements give breadth, firmness, and vigour to the bodily organs. Love diffuses through the mind warmth, enthusiasm, energy, the elements of genius, and gives an inexpressible charm to the feelings of the heart. All that is brave, noble, generous, heroic, and all that is sweet, voluptuous, tender, and endearing, spring from the influence or the sentiment of love.

When this sentiment is undeveloped, when the cerebellum is small and inactive, and when the generative organs are lacking in energy, the whole character suffers. It is cold, heartless, selfish, unfeeling, and wanting in the generous impulses and enthusiasm. And whatever be the cause of this lack of development or activity, the effects are nearly the same, and afford the most convincing proofs of what we have stated to be the proper influence of this wonderful faculty. If the development of the cerebellum is checked by the removal of the testicles in the male, or the ovaries in the female, at an early age, we have the most striking results. In the male, the beard does not grow, nor the hair upon the pubes. The larynx does not expand, and the voice retains the high treble

Or contralto pitch of boyhood. The operation of castration was formerly employed in Italy for this purpose. The muscles remain soft, and there is a tendency to fatness and effeminacy in the whole aspect. The mental and moral character is of a corresponding emasculation. There is feebleness, coldness, selfishness, cowardice, and a general lack of all we convey by the word manhood.

Now, similar effects are produced by early habits of masturbation, or self-abuse, and also by early excesses in sexual indulgence.

The effects of a similar check of development upon the female are equally remarkable ; but, in some respects, the reverse of the above. Love, that makes men manly, makes women womanly. Where there is destruction of the ovaries, or arrest of development, either of the ovaries or the cerebellum in girls, they grow large and coarse. The pelvis does not expand. The hair upon the pubes is thin and straggling ; the bosom remains flat ; a thin beard covers the chin ; not the rich down that sometimes gives a more voluptuous softness to the female lip, but a scraggy, straggling, half masculine beard; the voice becomes rough and masculine, and the whole appearance is that of an ambiguous being, neither male nor female, but partaking of the nature of each. The character, also, is cold, repulsive, rude, selfish, and cruel : the reverse of the truly feminine nature.

And in woman, as in man, similar effects are produced by any arrest of the development, or any exhaustion of the sentiment and organism of love ; but excess, which exhausts the other powers, and disturbs the harmony of the system, may only produce great and diseased activity of Amativeness ; when we have different effects from those which attend upon its destruction.

There can be no more powerful illustration of the

proper influence of the generative function over the animal and organic systems than those we have just given, and we have such illustrations, in a greater or less degree, all around us. No nature can be blessed with any quality so noble and ennobling as a healthy development of the principle of love. No nature can be so cursed as by its destruction or deprivation. All that is great, and noble, and beautiful in human character or capacity, or destiny, rests upon this basis. All that is base, and mean, and miserable, may find its source in the want, or disease, or perversion of this principle.

And the first effects, as I have said, of this influence are, as I believe, intended to be shown in the development of the individual, and not in the continuation of the species. The nervous power that is generated in the cerebellum, in man, and which is expended in the production of zoosperms in the testes, if not exhausted in their expulsion, and by their loss, is thrown back into the system, and strengthens every part. It is a fountain of life and energy; a vital force, which acts in every direction; a motive power, which infuses manhood into every organ of the brain and every fibre of the body. It is like the vital heat that warms the whole body, and then warms bodies around us, and which must not be exhausted.

Nature, under favourable conditions, has provided for this mode of action. Youth is the season of enterprise and action. The constitution is developed by hardy exercises, and the mind by studies. There is a restless and eager desire for knowledge and variety of occupation. And love is yet more romantic than passionate, more ideal than actual. It dwells in the imagination, and should not descend into the senses. So the nervous power, generated in the cerebellum— the divine energy that reigns in the soul—perfects the whole nature, and thus fits it for the mature accomplishment of its final object.

And in woman, while the organic action of the ovaries goes on, in the production, ripening, and throwing off of germs; if there is no expenditure of nervous force in sexual pleasure, no fecundation of the ovum, and consequently no evolution of the fœtus, her vital force is also expended in mental and physical development, and in fitting her for the functions of love and maternity, for which she is not well prepared until the accumulation and action of this force has brought to her a certain degree of maturity. The early germs in woman are less fitted for fecundation than those which appear later; and the zoosperms which are produced by the male in the first years of puberty, have less power in the production of healthy offspring. There is no doubt that the first activity of the generative function should be expended in energising the individual rather than in the propagation of the species.

The passion of love, or the propensity of Amativeness, varies in the sexes, and in individuals of each sex. No two persons look alike; no two feel alike, nor, unless under compulsion, can they act alike. They may act in harmony; but harmony is not unison. Where we can find two persons in the world with the same form, features, and expression, the same development of faculties, in the same proportions and relations, we may expect them to feel and act alike, and be governed by the same rules.

In certain respects all men are alike; but their likeness is consistent with an infinite individuality. In certain respects the faculties and passions of different individuals are alike; but in others they very notably differ. How varied are the tastes and capacities connected with the organ of Tune! One person can only understand the simplest melody; others revel in complicated harmonies. Alimentiveness in one man tends to the desire of a single delicacy; another seems omnivorous. In Art one is fond of portraits, another of landscapes; one delights in the simple and severe, another loves the ornate and luxurious. Observe the various tastes in dress, when fashion does not compel everybody to follow a particular standard. In religion, in ambition, in pride, in friendship, in all faculties, sentiments, and passions, we have these varieties of individuality, necessary to the perfection of social harmony. Shall we deny to the great passion of love, and the great function of generation, the same individuality and the same variety?

The passion of love, as it reigns in the soul of man, harmonising and energising his animal and organic systems, has three general modes of expression.

1. It gives a feeling of regard for the whole opposite sex. It inspires in man a gallant respect for woman; in woman, a tender regard for man.

2. In a circumscribed sphere, it is social in its character and action. A man has for the women of his acquaintance, whom he meets in society, and with whom he is on terms of kindly familiarity, a very different feeling from any he entertains towards the other sex. Women and men, with no bond of personal love, still have a more cordial feeling toward each other, than they commonly have toward persons of their own sex. This is seen in families, in society, and in schools where both sexes mix freely together. But under the customary repressions of fashion, and opinion, and puritanism, we find men and women driven into false and unnatural connections with those of their own sex —yet even here we see masculine natures attaching themselves to feminine, and everywhere the action of the great physical and moral law—unlike natures attract each other—like natures repel.

3. Personal love, beginning with a spiritual attraction, becoming voluptuous desire and seeking its ultimate expression in sexual union. This is the last, fullest, and most perfect action of the amative passion;

that which consummates the life and happiness of the individual, and governs the destiny of the race.

Reproduction in the vegetable world is, in the higher organisations, as distinctly a sexual process as among animals; and in the flowers, or sexual organs of plants, we have a great variety of relations, from the union of a single stamen and pistil, of a pistil with two, three, four, or almost any number of stamens, or several pistils receiving their pollen indiscriminately from a number of stamens. Vegetables are monogamic, polygamic, and polyandrous. (See any work on botany, or read Darwin's "Loves of the Plants.")

In animals, again, we have all varieties of sexual relations. Some are entirely promiscuous, any male fecundating any female. Then we have the polygamic relations which exist among fowls, seals, and other gregarious animals, in which one male has a harem of several females, who are made his by his own attraction, or the right of the strongest. On the other hand, we see female animals, especially those who produce several young at a litter, receiving successively the embraces of several males. The queen bee, the only perfect female in the hive, has for her service two or three hundred drones, whose sole office is the fecundation of the eggs, which are to produce her numerous offspring. On the other hand, one ram is sufficient for a large flock of sheep, one bull for a herd of cows, and one stallion for a number of mares.

Many animals, however, are monogamic. Most of our birds copulate in pairs, and are capable of ardent and exclusive affections. Elephants are found both in pairs and in herds; monkeys pair, but are not exclusive in their amours. The wolves seek each other only once a-year, and cohabit promiscuously. The only one of all the species of deer that is constant, is the roebuck. An abundance of facts, to be found in any good work on natural history, illustrate the varieties of this action of love in the animal races.

In the human species, the love relation exists in such variety as might seem to indicate, what many believe, that man includes in himself the nature of all the lower animals. In the early ages, and what are called the patriarchal times, polygamy seems to have been the unquestioned practice. It is now tolerated by law or custom over three-fourths of the world, and is practiced to a great extent over the other fourth.

Polyandrous relations, or the union of one woman to several men, under the sanction of law or custom, is more rare; but there are not wanting examples of this. In Thibet, in Malabar, in the South Sea islands, it is allowed to a woman to have two or more husbands; and, in point of fact, this is practiced to some extent over the civilised world. In some of the most polite countries in Europe, custom has sanctioned women of the higher classes having a lover as well as a husband; and such relations exist, and are more or less tolerated everywhere, while men are still more free in their ideas, and promiscuous in their indulgences.

If we examine the society around us, we shall find persons of varied creeds and practices in the sexual relations.

1. Strict monogamists, who believe in a single love, which endures through all time and all eternity. This belief does not admit of one love succeeding another, much less two at the same time. A second love is profanity, a second marriage adultery. Yet persons zealously avowing this belief, are found engaging in a succession of amours. Their excuse is, that in each case they have been mistaken. The person supposed to be the true conjugial partner, the heaven-appointed mate, proved not to be the right one. They have nothing to do but to go on trying, atoning for each

successive adultery, by their efforts to find a true relation.

2. Moderate monogamists, who allow of a succession of love relations, but do not admit of but one at a time. This is the ordinary view of marriage, in which the bond can only be dissolved by the death of one of the parties; or by such an outrage against the relation as is equivalent to death, such as adultery.

3. There are those who believe in a central or pivotal love, transcending, and perhaps outlasting all others; but around which may revolve other loves, affections, or fancies, not inconsistent, but entirely harmonious with, the prime and pivotal relation.

Observation shows us that there are men capable of a single love, whose intensity absorbs and exhausts their whole passional nature, and the same is probably oftener the case with women. This is the love we read about in poems and novels, but see rather less of in real life.

Men who have romantic fancies in boyhood and early youth, and violent love fits in early manhood, which give place to calmer, stronger, and more enduring loves in their maturity, may be exclusive or monogamic; or, with more varied and expansive natures, strong loves may be consistent with subordinate affections, desires, and gratifications. These differences in exclusive intensity, or expansive variety, extend to the whole character, and a man or woman of a wide range of capacity or genius, who is capable of alternations, and even of doing many things at the same time, may be expected to have a like capacity in love.

Men who combine weakness with versatility; who go equally in every direction, but strongly in none, are likely to be unsettled and promiscuous, either to change continually, or to have a disorderly variety. These are not pivotal characters, nor are they capable of an exclusive attachment. In this latter class, we have a vast number of men, and not a few women.

Theoretically, in Christian states, the monogamic principle of the union of a single pair for life is adopted; but this principle is widely violated in practice. This monogamic union is the legal marriage, from which, in some countries, there is no divorce; in others, divorce is allowed on the ground of adultery, and, in some states, for desertion, ill-treatment, drunkenness, and various causes.

Marriage, according to the common acceptation, is the legal union of a man and woman, who, from any motive, have agreed to live together in exclusive cohabitation. Adultery is the violation of this compact by either party.

Marriage, in a higher and purer sense, is the union of two persons in mutual love; and adultery is, perhaps, best defined as any gratification of mere lust, or the sensual nature, without the sanctification of a true love, and apart from the lawful uses of marriage. According to these definitions, a true marriage may be what the laws call adultery, while the real adultery is an unloving marriage.

The Catholic Church teaches that marriage is a sacrament, and therefore it does not permit divorce, but only separation; neither party being allowed to marry again until the death of the other. It is literally "until death do us part."

In plants there is but one act of impregnation, by a single organ, which occurs at what may be called its season of puberty. Its office performed, the useless organs wither. The whole flower drops off, when its function has been performed. Some plants produce but one set of generative organs, and then the whole plant perishes. These are the annuals. Others go on producing flowers and buds year after year. These are the perennials.

There are many of the lower varieties of animals which perform but a single act of generation, and then die. The higher animals continue the process through many years. As a general rule, the lower the animal in the scale, the more prolific. A fish produces millions of eggs ; the higher mammalia seldom have more than one at a birth. Some breed in litters every few weeks ; others require two or three years to produce and suckle a single offspring.

In the females of most animals, there occurs a period in which they are ready to receive and solicit the embraces of the male. This is called the period of heat, or the rutting season. It is that in which the ova are ripened, and cast off from the ovaries, and when the sexual congress is demanded for their impregnation. This period, which in animals is more or less frequent, according to their periods of gestation, corresponds to the periodic menstrual evacuation in the human female.

The males of animals differ with respect to their readiness for the performance of their part in the sexual function. In some, the feeling seems not to exist in the intervals, and the testicles are shrunk and inactive ; but when the rutting season of the female arrives, as it usually does in the spring, these organs enlarge, secrete with vigour, and the animals seem filled with a fury of desire. The stag, usually gentle, is at this time fierce and dangerous ; but in animals where the periods are frequent, or where one male encounters many females, the organs are always in an active condition, and the male always ready to perform the duties which nature has imposed upon him, and to enjoy the pleasures which she gives as a reward. But it must not be supposed that pleasure is the only attraction. The instinct of reproduction is above all mere sensual gratification. It is by no means certain that this act is always one of pleasure to animals, while, in our own species, the sexual congress is often to the woman either entirely

H

indifferent, or painful.   Gestation is to many a long disease, and parturition a death agony.   Still, the desire for offspring triumphs over these terrible perversions.

In animals where there is but one gestation in a year, there is usually but one period of heat; but while the periods of gestation and lactation extend over nearly two years in the human female; when these are at an end, she regularly, every month, throws off an ovum, marked by the menstrual discharge; and, of course, is every month prepared to receive the sexual embrace.   It seems to be fairly inferable, that once a month is the natural period in which a woman requires sexual union; and it may be doubted whether any greater frequency is not a violation of natural law.   At this period, however, when in a healthy condition, she is full of ardour, has a great capacity for enjoyment, and is seldom satisfied with a single sexual act.   The period of excitement, moreover, may last for several days, or all the time the ovum is passing from the ovary to the uterus.   Once there, it should not be disturbed by any amative excitement, whose tendency from that time forward, is to produce abortion.   It is the law of all nature; a law that is said never to be violated even among savages, out of Christendom, that there should be no sexual union during gestation.   It is not permitted among animals, and over three quarters of the world is looked upon as infamous in our own species.   It is also inconsistent with the performance of the function of lactation or nursing ; and no woman, mother or wet nurse, who gives milk to a child, should be subjected to sexual intercourse.   This is one reason why women, who do not nurse their children, because their husbands will not refrain from sexual indulgence, try to get unmarried mothers as wet nurses for their babes.

And sexual intercourse during pregnancy is a dis turbance of that function and an injury to mother and child, especially if the female partakes in its enjoyment. It is the most common cause of abortion and miscarriage. and increases the pain and danger of childbirth. No woman naturally seeks union at such period : no woman can safely submit to it. What should we think of any animal but man, which should do as he does in these matters? I see no physiological reason why a woman should desire sexual union, after pregnancy, until her next menstrual period, which will not normally take place until she has finished nursing.

Man differs very materially from woman in the exercise of the procreative function. From the age of puberty, the action of the testes is uninterrupted. I can find no hint of periodicity, unless it has been created by habit. Whatever restrains he may have, must be moral; for they are not physical like woman's. And while, in woman, the production of ova ceases at from forty-five to fifty-five, the activity of the organs in man continues, and he is capable of generating until a late period of life, and in some cases when more than a century old. Man has no function corresponding in periodicity to menstruation ; no diversions of the vital forces engaged in this function, like those of pregnancy and lactation. But in this function man must be governed by the requirements of natural law, which is the basis of morality. And the law is that he should respond to the feminine requirement, and never go beyond it. This is the law throughout the animal creation, and to it man is no exception. Woman was not made to be a harlot for man, the instrument of his pleasures, in marriage or out of it. Sexual union is for birth, and to be had when the pure, unperverted feminine instinct demands it; never for mere sensual gratification, and assuredly never when it may defeat the very end it was intended to accomplish.

The influence of the organ of Amativeness stimulates the action of the secreting or sperm-preparing organs, the testicles.   The presence of the seminal fluid in the seminal vesicles, re-acts upon the brain, and the mind glows with voluptuous ideas.   Under their influence, men are gallant, kind, attentive, and loving to women; ever seeking their favours; ever pressing their suit.   It is the part of woman to accept or repulse; to grant or refuse.   It is her right to reign a passional queen; to say, " thus far shalt thou come, and no farther."   It is for her nature to decide both as to whom she will admit to her embraces, and when; and there is no despotism upon this earth like that which compels a woman to the embraces of a man she does not love; or to receive the embraces of a man she does love when her nature does not require them, and when she cannot partake in the sexual embrace without injury to herself and danger to her offspring.   If a woman has any right in this world, it is the right to herself; and if there is anything in this world she has a right to decide, it is who shall be the father of her children. She has an equal right to decide whether she will have children, and to choose the time for having them.

This is a law of nature, respected throughout the animal kingdom.   The female everywhere refuses sexual union with the male, except at the appointed season; and compulsion at any time, and especially during pregnancy, cannot be called beastly, for this would be a libel on the brutes.

The expressions of love antecedent to, and connected with its ultimation, are varied and beautiful, involving the whole being.   Love gives light, and a trembling suffusion to the eye, a soft, tremulous tenderness to the voice, a sweet sadness to the demeanour, or a deep joyousness; a certain warmth and voluptuousness preside over the movements of the body; blushes come often to the cheeks, and the eyes are cast down with consciousness; the heart swells, and beats tumultuously; there is a radiant idealisation of the beloved object, who seems to enamoured eyes clothed with every perfection; an exquisite delight pervades the sense of feeling; every touch, even of the garments, gives pleasure to those who love; hands are clasped with a thrill of delight; lips meet in rapturous kisses; and the same instinctive attraction, which brings together the two sexes of the lower animals, acts not less powerfully in man; but should act always under the influence of tender sentiment, refined feeling, reason and conscience, for the greatest good as well as the highest happiness. This sexual congress, should, for the protection of all concerned, have the sanction of needful social regulations.

There are a few practical observations, which may be properly made here, connected with the physiology of the sexual congress. The organs of generation, in both sexes, are excited and stimulated by idleness, luxury, and every form of voluptuousness. Where it is desirable to avoid such excitement, all these must be guarded against. Passionate poetry and romances, warm pictures, dancing, especially the dancing of the stage, the fashionable display of female arms and bosoms, all fond toyings, and personal freedoms between the sexes, must be avoided by those with whom chastity is a necessity of age or circumstance. The lips are supplied with nerves of sensation from the cerebellum; and the kisses of the lips are sacred to love. The bosom is also supplied with nerves from the same source, and it is in the most direct and intimate sympathy with the female generative organs. A woman of sensibility, who would preserve her chastity, must guard her bosom well.

But the best safeguard against one passion, is to arouse another, and, if possible, many others. Friendship is often a safeguard against love; even the friendship of young persons of opposite sexes. In the family, in schools, and in society, the more a friendly familiarity exists, the less likelihood is there of amative excitement and indulgence. Friendship comes so near to love, in its character, that it often takes its place, and is sometimes mistaken for it. Business, study, active exercises, amusement, ambition, reverence, a constant occupation of mind and body, divert the vital forces into so many channels, that the system feels no pressing wants in this direction, and men live in the bustle of active life, for months and even years, without amative wants.

Women govern themselves much more easily than men. With great numbers, continence is no virtue, for they have not the least attraction for sexual connection, nor are they capable of sexual enjoyment. This is, indeed, a diseased condition, hereditary or acquired; but it is common to an incredible degree. But even with women of passionate natures, who are capable of the most ardent love, and the fullest enjoyment, certain conditions are necessary to the awakening of sexual desire. They must love, and be beloved. Love must begin in the soul as a sentiment, come down into the heart as a passion, before it can descend into the body as a desire. Such a woman will be continent without the least difficulty, so long as she does not love; but when she loves a man, she gives herself to him, soul and body. Happy the man who can inspire and respond to such a love! Happy the child born of such a union! Happy the human race when there shall be no others!

CHAPTER VIII.

IMPREGNATION.

THE formation of the zoosperm, or seminal animal-cule, in man, and the ovum in woman, belongs to the domain of organic life, yet all the highest powers of the soul, and the soul's organs, are engaged in the work. For there is to be more than a mere bodily organisation formed—a mass of bone, muscle, and various tissues. First of all, there is to be generated an immortal soul.

The soul of man, like his body, is the creation of Infinite Wisdom and Power, but God works by means and in accordance with fixed laws; and as bodies are so formed as to generate other bodies, so it may be that souls, in like manner, generate souls. This may be the mode chosen by the Creator; so that the parents of every child are the parents of its immortal part, as well as its mortal. If souls were made apart, and then came into bodies formed for them, how could they be affected with what theologians call original sin—the evident depravity which exists in man, and so widely distinguishes him from all other creatures?

It is, in fact, the soul, so generated, if we accept the hypothesis to which analogy points, which forms the body which, for some years, is to be its habitation, the medium of its perceptions, and the instrument of its expression. The generation of souls seems necessary, indeed, to explain the facts of the hereditary transmission of moral and mental, as well as physical qualities. The souls of children—their moral characters—are like those of their parents, and compounded of those of their fathers and mothers, some more resembling one, some the other. We never find the soul of a European in the body of a Hottentot, or the soul of a North American Indian in the body of a native of China.

All varieties of human character are expressed in differences of organisation. The physiologist reads them in temperament and general conformation; the physiognomist sees them written in the lines of the face; the phrenologist in the developments of the brain; but all these are effects, not causes. It is not the body that shapes the soul, but the soul that forms the body. It is the brain that gives shape to the skull, and not the skull that circumscribes the brain's development. It is the faculty that shapes the organ, and not the organ that hampers the faculty. The soul forms the cortical substance of the brain, and from this the whole nervous system; and it is the nervous system, acting upon the blood, that builds up the whole body, and not, by any means, the reverse of this.

Two human beings, uniting as one, becoming "one flesh," have thus given to them the power, or are the appointed instruments, of generating a third being— body, soul, and spirit. They form it according to their own capacities. Or, if the soul have any other origin it must be admitted that they limit its expression and development, and all its earthly manifestation; so that there are great and little souls, beautiful and ugly souls; and so on of all varieties of human character.

But it must also be admitted that there are facts of human intelligence and goodness not easily accounted for upon the theory of hereditary transmission. How came a Shakespeare to spring up in Warwickshire? What do we know of the progenitors of our greatest geniuses in every department of human achievement? We must admit of other influences — of supernal inspirations.

It may be that if we could know the conditions and peculiar relations and elevations of the souls of parents in the generation of souls of genius, we might see a solution of the mystery. But leaving out such apparently exceptional facts, we can see that, as a general rule, in families, nations, and races, the children resemble their parents. English, Scottish, Welsh, Irish, have peculiarities as marked as Chinese, Negroes, North American Indians, and Esquimaux.

And the soul grows like as the body grows, and changes as the body changes, and grows strong by exercise, and great by the reception of soul nutriment; and is prepared to generate still higher souls: and this is the law of education, development, progress. So we have diseases of the soul as of the body; these re-acting on each other; and each susceptible of proper curative treatment. Does not the mind feed on thoughts and feelings, and get starved or surfeited, and grow dyspeptic on trash or sweetmeats, or exhilarated and intoxicated? Who has not felt his whole soul strengthened by communion with some strong spirit?

This sublime function of the generation of human beings, soul and body, is performed by the two male and female organs, the testes and the ovaries, acted upon by every human faculty, and modified by every human circumstance and action.

It is not in my power to solve the questions respecting the portions of the mental and physical organisation, contributed by either parent. I see no reason to believe in any such partition. I think each has a share in the formation of every part, though in any part the influence of one or the other may preponderate. A child may resemble either of its parents, or both, or it may be more like one of its grandparents than either. It may have more of the mind of one, or the physical constitution of the other, or both may be evenly mingled. If a man have a powerfully-developed and active mind, and a woman a vigorous organic system, it is likely that their child will resemble each in their strongest points. Germ cell and sperm cell, I believe, are both engaged in the formation of every faculty and organ.

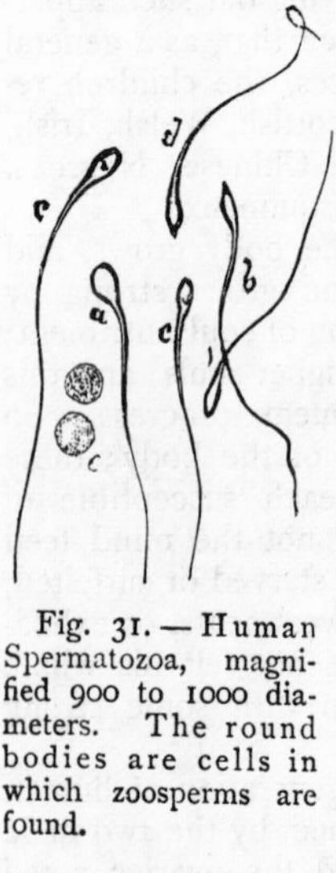

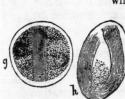

Fig. 31. — Human Spermatozoa, magnified 900 to 1000 diameters. The round bodies are cells in which zoosperms are found.

The sperm cell is the result of the action of that complex organ, the testicle—an organ composed of a vast surface of tubular structure, and amply supplied with nerve and blood, by which, and out of which, these animate cells are formed. Then, within the primitive sperm cell, appear cells, and within these are formed, first in a circular mass, a great number of exceedingly minute living beings, consisting of an oval-shaped body, and a long tail. This self-propelling cell swims in a fluid substance, like the white of an egg, but more opaque, formed partly in the testes, and partly secreted by the prostate gland. In full health and vigour, these zoosperms are very numerous and active; in sickness or exhaustion they are few and weak, and in certain states of the system they entirely disappear, and the power of fecundation no longer exists. The primitive germ cell first bursts, setting free the smaller cells, and

Fig. 32.—Evolution of Spermatozoa.

these, in turn, liquefy, and set free the now perfected zoosperms; the seminal fluid containing them then passes on through the vasa deferentia, up the spermatic cord, passes through the walls of the abdomen, and is received, with the prostatic fluid, according to the common belief, into the seminal vesicles, which are a reservoir in which it is retained, until expelled by the action of the proper muscular apparatus in the sexual orgasm.

The zoosperms retain their power of motion, under favourable circumstances, for hours, and even days, after being ejected. In fish, which do not copulate, they swim about in the water, until they come in contact with the eggs spawned by the female. The ripe eggs, or hard roe, may be taken from the body of a female fish, and the testicle, or soft roe, from the male, and fecundation produced by mingling them together, and ponds and rivers may be stocked with fish, by this mode of artificial impregnation.

In the generation of mammalia, by the entrance of the penis into the vagina, the spermatic fluid should be thrown into the mouth of the uterus, and then, by the contractions of that organ, forced up the fallopian tubes, toward the ovaries. But several circumstances may prevent this being accomplished. The male organ may be too short to reach the uterus; it may not, from some malformation, be even able to effect an entrance into the vagina, and still impregnation may take place; for the active zoosperms, in great numbers, move every way with a rapid motion, and are able to find their way through the entire length of vagina, uterus, and fallopian tubes. On the other hand, when the womb is too low, in the common ailment of falling of the womb, the semen may pass beyond the mouth of the womb, and be lodged in a deep fold of the vagina, which may prevent impregnation.

While the testicles are engaged in the evolution of
zoosperms, the ovaries of the female are no less active
in forming and ripening the ova; but with this striking
difference, that, while zoosperms are formed by millions, and may be ejected day after day, we have but
one or two, or in rare cases, from three to five, ova
perfected once a month; and this process ceases during
gestation, and should also be suspended during lactation.   The ovum, or egg, which, in all its essential
parts, is alike in all animals, and which consists of a
cell, a nucleus, and a nucleolus, is found in the stroma
or mass of the ovary.   The egg of the common fowl
may be taken as the type of all eggs.   Its yolk and
white are of immense bulk, compared with its germinal
spot, because there must be contained within the shell
the entire matter of which the perfect chicken is formed.
In the human ovum this matter is small in quantity, as
the fœtus, from an early period, is nourished by the
blood of the mother in the uterus.

When this egg is fully formed, ripened, or matured.
the cell which envelopes it swells, bursts, and sets it
free.   It is then grasped by the fimbriated extremity
of the fallopian tube, and begins its journey down that
passage to the uterus.   It may be impregnated at any
time after it is set free by the bursting of the graafian
vesicle, until its arrival in the uterus, and possibly
until its expulsion from that receptacle.

It will be seen that conception can only take place
under certain well-defined circumstances.   First, there
must be a ripened ovum, set free from its graafian
vesicle.   This takes place regularly once a month,
after the period of puberty, and in all healthy females
is marked by the menstrual evacuation.   If this evacuation is coincident with the expulsion of the ovum from
the ovary, impregnation must take place, if at all,
within eight, or, at most, twelve days of that period.
The zoosperms may meet the ovum on its passage, or,

possibly, the ovum may find the zoosperm awaiting its arrival. It follows that sexual connection, to answer its natural end, should take place not more than three days before the beginning, or within ten days after the menstrual evacuation.

But in the diseases and irregularities of our lives, with the excitements of stimulating food and general false habits, with the continual over-excitement and exercise of the generative organs, these processes become irregular, and their normal signs not to be depended on. Ova may be prematurely ripened by excitement of the ovaries, caused by sexual indulgence. The menstrual evacuation, which degenerates into a real hemorrhage, becomes irregular and uncertain, as well as depraved in its character. Consequently, the rule that sexual union, to produce impregnation, must take place either immediately before, or a few days after, menstruation, admits of exceptions. It is a safe rule for those who desire to procreate; but not entirely safe for those who would avoid it, as many, for good reasons, may.

Menstruation appears to be a throwing off of the fluids concerned in the ripening and expulsion of the ova. In a perfectly healthy state, the menstrual fluid is very small in quantity, and scarcely tinged with the red colouring matter of the blood. In disease, it becomes a genuine hemorrhage, lasts for three or four days, or longer, with the loss of several ounces of blood, mingled with the proper menstrual fluid. There is no better test of the health of a woman than the one I have just given.

In what manner the actual impregnation of the ovum takes place, we have no positive knowledge. Microscopic observers assert that they have seen the zoosperm enter the ovum by an opening left for that purpose. It has even been fancied, that the body and tail of the seminal animalcule form the rudiments of the brain and spinal cord! Observations of the progress of fœtal development warrant no such conclusion. If it could be established, it would prove that the animal system of nerves was formed by the male parent, and the organic by the female. The resemblance of children to their parents, and all the phenomena of hereditary transmission of qualities, prove that both parents are concerned in the production of every part.

We have, then, two objects here of microscopic minuteness. One is the germinal point in the female ovum; the other is the zoosperm, or some portion of it. In each of these minute organisations is comprised the elements of a glorious and immortal being. Each contains, moreover, the rudiments of the very form and qualities of that being, physical, moral, and intellectual. There, in that point of matter, that pellucid cell, we have the shape and air, the talents and genius, the honesty or roguery, the pride or humility, the benevolence or selfishness of the future man. We have what determines the form of his head and hands, the contour of his nose and chin, the colour of his eyes and hair. Moreover, this spermatic animalcule, or this cell germ, has all hereditary idiosyncrasies and diseases, gout, scrofula, venereal taint, or insanity.

We can scarcely conceive of this, yet we must admit it. All the grand and energetic qualities that made a Cæsar or a Napoleon—all that can be fairly attributed to blood and birth, to hereditary influences, must have been contained in one or both these atoms.

I do not underrate the influences that may act upon the fœtus during gestation. I give full credit to the power of education in forming the human character; but I assert that all which makes the basis of the character, mental and physical, must reside in the germ and the spermatozoon, and must combine at the moment of impregnation, or the union of these principles.

For all the qualities of soul and body which make the differences between a mouse, a dog, a horse, an elephant, must be in their germinal principles. The appearance of the zoosperms in different animals varies slightly under the microscope—that of the ova scarcely at all. Moreover, when two nearly allied species of animals engender; when, for example, the zoosperm of the ass unites with the ovum of the mare, each parent is found to contribute to the mental and physical qualities of the offspring. In all crossings of different breeds of animals, we find the same effects produced, the more powerful impressing themselves most strongly, and the two sexes giving each certain peculiar characteristics.

Nor is this by any means less notably the fact in the human species. When sexual commerce takes place between a negro and a white woman, the child partakes of the mental and physical qualities of both.

If we do not understand the process by which the union of the male and female elements is accomplished, in the generation of the new being, the conditions under which it must take place are more clear to us. From a multitude of observations, it appears,—

1. That the ovum, in a state of healthy maturity, must have been set free from the ovary. This is not the case with some of the lower animals. There are insects, in whom a single act of the male will fecundate successive generations. In birds, the male principle seems to be added before the egg is mature.

2. The sperma must be recent, and must contain living, active zoosperms.

3. The smallest quantity, and probably a single zoosperm, is sufficient, if it comes in contact with the ovum.

4. It is not necessary that there should be any enjoyment of coition, on the part of the female. Women

who have none, seem even more prolific than others. It may take place in sleep, or other insensibility. In men, also, the orgasm may be accompanied with no pleasure, and even with pain.

5. Even the sexual union is not indispensable. There is no doubt that a female ovum may be impregnated by semen conveyed to it artificially; and a woman, if she chose, might have a child without ever coming into personal contact with a man. This has been shown in animals by abundant experiments, and is said to have occurred in human subjects. There is, however, not the slightest reason to doubt the result, if the experiment were fairly tried.

There are a few other points of interest, which may as well be discussed here as elsewhere. Few questions are of more practical importance to the human race than under what circumstances the generative act should be performed. I will give my opinion briefly, stating the reasons where they are not self-evident or apparent.

1. The generative act should be performed by two persons arrived at a full development of their powers, physical and intellectual. The children of young and immature parents are apt to be weak and scrofulous. Age cannot be given as an absolute index of maturity, and there are some who are never mature.

2. It should be performed with all the attraction and charm of a mutual love; and the existence of this is the best evidence that the parties are suitably related to each other; for those similarities of constitution, which forbid the marriage of near relations, and which often exist without consanguinity, and are sometimes wanting with it, also prevent a true love. Hence, marriages of family interest, convenience, similarity of tastes, and friendship, may be very unfortunate with respect to children. Love, and its functions, require a mingling of opposite qualities.

No man ought ever to beget a child for a woman he does not love; and, especially, no woman ought ever to submit to the sexual embrace of a man, unless assured that the union is sanctioned by a mutual affec· tion.

3. It should not be performed, by man or woman, so as to entail hereditary disease upon their offspring. Insanity, scrofula, consumption, syphilis, diseased amativeness, deformities of body, or distressing singularities of mind, should not be entailed upon posterity.

4. A woman should avoid conception, if her pelvis is so small, or so deformed, as to hazard her own life in delivery, or destroy that of the child, or compel an abortion.

5. In the present social state, men and women should refrain from having children, unless they see a reasonable prospect of giving them suitable nurture and education. We have no right to inflict an injury upon an individual or society.

But how is pregnancy to be prevented? There is one way that is natural, simple, and effectual. It is to refrain from the sexual act. It is easily done by most women, and by many men. In every civilised community, thousands live in celibacy, many from necessity, many from choice. In England and the older American States, there is a large surplus female population. In catholic countries the whole priesthood, and great numbers of religious, of both sexes, take vows of perpetual chastity. This practice has existed for at least sixteen centuries.

I have shown that, in ordinary cases, conception can only take place when connection is had a day or two before, or ten, or, for safety's sake, say sixteen days after menstruation. There is, then, a fortnight each month, when the female is not liable to impregnation; but it must be remembered, that if she is amatively excited in this interval, the ripening of

I

the ova may be hastened, and the very result precipi-
tated that it is intended to avoid. And it is also to
be observed, that the natural period for sexual union is
when it is demanded for the purpose of procreation,
and that the use of marriage, or the sexual act, for
mere pleasure, and using any means to avoid impregnation, are unnatural. It is questionable, therefore,
whether we can morally justify the use of any means
to prevent conception. If it can ever be justified, it
is when a woman is unwillingly compelled to submit
to the embraces of her husband, while her health or
other conditions forbid her to have children.

The limitation of the number of children is advocated
as a right and a duty by a class of social reformers, who,
at the same time, insist upon the right and even duty
of frequent gratification of the amative propensities by
all persons who have arrived at the age of puberty.
Virtue, chastity, continence, they denounce as unnatural and mischievous. I hold, on the contrary, that
the law of a pure and unperverted nature, is the law
of chastity, and that it is consistent with the highest
health, and the best bodily, mental, and moral condition of men and women; and that men and women
can and ought to be as natural and moral, at least, as
the lower orders of the animal creation.

The secularist philanthropists who teach in several
languages and many editions of their favourite book,
that it is not only the right, but the duty, of all persons, married or single, from the age of puberty, to
have frequent and regular exercise of amativeness;
who hold that what good men in all ages have called
virtue is a vice, that chastity is wickedness and continence criminality, and that lewdness, fornication,
and adultery are moral duties, are obliged also to
advocate the use of preventive checks to an increase
of population. Openly advocating universal prostitution, concubinage, and promiscuity, with its

unavoidable incests and demoralization; seeking for sensual pleasure rather than the true purposes of the sexual relation; wishing to enjoy a selfish gratification and to avoid the burthens and responsibilities which naturally belong to it, they teach that it is the right and duty of men and women to prevent pregnancy.

Every mode of prevention, other than that of living in chastity, is an evident violation of nature, and can only be resorted to as a choice between unavoidable evils.   Pressure upon the urethra causes disease; withdrawal is little better than masturbation—the sin of Onan.   The very thought and intention of enjoying a natural pleasure and at the same time doing something to hinder the natural effect of such enjoyment, is a source of evil.   The soul participates in the act and the enjoyment; but when pleasure is divorced from the natural motive and use, it becomes a mere sensual gratification, against which conscience protests and even instinct revolts.   Our only safety, and our highest good, in this as in all things, is in finding what is true, natural, and therefore in accordance with the law of life written in our moral and physical constitution.   This is the path of health, purity. and happiness.

CHAPTER IX.

MORALS OF THE SEXUAL RELATION.

HERE, as well as anywhere, I may say what may usefully be said on sexual morality, and of what it seems well for every one to know of what we may call the ethics of the sexual relation.

From birth to puberty, or the period when the sexual organs assume their natural functions, which is at the age of about seventeen in males and fifteen in females, with variations of a year or two, over and under,—during the period of infancy and adolescence, there should be no excitement, no irritation, no action of any kind in the amative system; but perfect purity in thought, and word, and deed.

It would be well if children had no sensation and no idea of sex. Unfortunately, the exciting and diseasing habits of civilisation tend to produce an unhealthy precocity in the young of both sexes. Children either fall into habits of solitary vice—from hereditary predisposition, or a stimulating diet, — or they are taught libidinous and destructive practices by ignorant or unprincipled servants, or companions or schoolfellows who have been in some way corrupted.

If they could be kept in ignorance and innocence, it might be best—but the risk of trying to do so is so great, that it seems to me better that every child should be taught, as early as it has the power to sin and the liability to suffer, what is the sin against nature it has to avoid. It is a terrible thing that the whole life of a beautiful boy or girl should be wrecked, because, in pure ignorance, he or she falls into a bad habit spontaneously, or is taught it by another. Surely it would be better if every child were clearly told and solemnly warned of its danger. Of the practice of masturbation, and its terrible consequences, more will be found in the chapters on disease.

With the period of puberty, sometimes before, comes the season of sentimental love. And this love should be kept entirely free from the physical or reproductive element. Pure love is chastening and refining in its influence. It is imaginative, poetical, tender, romantic, heroic; and the longer this period lasts the better. As marriage should not take place until the bodily powers are considerably matured, there should not be in early love any desire or even thought of sexual union. The law of the purest and highest life is perfect purity, complete chastity, entire continence, before marriage. Society rigorously insists upon this with respect to women. Every man wishes his bride to come to his arms a virgin; but the law of nature is the same for both sexes. All women have an equal right to marry —all should come purely to the marriage bed. If young men are to have a license denied to young women, what are the means? Either adultery, which is such a crime that men justify the husband who kills both wife and paramour; or the seduction, ruin, and prostitution of unmarried women.

What is right for one sex must be right for both; what is wrong for one must be wrong for both. There can be no right of men to destroy a certain number of women, making them the victims of their lusts, in order that those they marry may be virtuous. We must either stand upon the Christian rule of sexual morality, or admit of universal license. We must have chaste youth and virtuous manhood and womanhood, or see our social world become one vast brothel of unbridled lust.

The law of married life is one of temperance or moderation—a natural use of marriage for its chief object, the begetting of offspring. The law of the whole animal world is sexual connection for the purpose of reproduction, only at such times and in such quantity as best favours that result. The females of all the animal races, insects, birds, beasts, in this matter govern, and admit the access of males only when they require it for the fecundation of germs and the production of offspring. They sternly refuse at all other times, and we should detest any animal that made pleasure alone the motive of sexual union. There can be no doubt that this is also the natural and healthful law of the human species.

The germs, as we have seen, are ripened and thrown off once a month. This, then, is the natural period of the sexual congress. It should take place when both parties are in full vigour—never in fatigue, never when exhausted by bodily or mental toil, never in sickness; above all, never when intoxicated. Body and mind should be free from all excitement but that of love, from all perturbation but that of a healthy desire. The condition of both parents at this period affects that of their offspring. There should be no excess, no exhaustion. The act should never be more than twice or thrice repeated, awaiting the result; and the congress should not be renewed until the next monthly period. If the menses do not appear, it is a sign that conception has taken place, and the expectant mother must then be sacred from all approach or the least amative excitement through the whole period of pregnancy and nursing. This law is respected by savages, and is regarded over a large part of the civilised world, and should never be violated. No breeder of horses, or cattle, or animals of any kind, would permit intercourse while they were with young—and the human female should assuredly be held as sacred.

A word of advice is needed for the young. The first union—the consummation of marriage—needs great care. The bride a man takes to his heart should be treated with exceeding delicacy. There should be no word or act to shock her modesty. The lover who has become a husband should be sober, discreet, and very careful to do her no injury. He can wait. It is a great happiness to wait, and to ask nothing until she is willing to grant him all. And in the embrace in which all is given, there must still be great care not to hurt, nor to injure a delicate organism. The vagina may be contracted—give it time to expand. The hymen may not readily yield—do not rupture it too rudely. Wait until the pleasure shall overcome the pain. Leave it

in good part to her own effort.   And in all this intercourse, if one would preserve its bloom and sweetness,
there should be the same tenderness, the same delicacy, the same unselfish regard for the happiness of
the other.   The best writer on this whole subject of
marriage is St. Paul, and his luminous epistles I commend to every reader.   In an honest and true love
there is no cause and no room for jealously.   "Perfect
love casteth out fear."

The power of producing germs in the ovaries, which
by fecundation develope into offspring, begins in woman
with, or in some cases even before, menstruation, and
continues to the "turn of life," or the period when it
ceases, usually at from forty-five to fifty-five years of
age.   Men have the power of procreation sometimes
to a very advanced age, and some have begotten
children when more than a hundred years old.   But
this power should be used with great care and temperance by the aged; and those who would live long,
and keep the energies of their bodies and minds, do
well to refrain from it altogether.   After fifty, sexual
pleasures are very exhausting.   They often bring on
paralysis or apoplexy.   The strongest old men are
celebates, or those who live in perfect continence.   A
woman who wishes to guard the health and life of
her husband, must induce him to entirely refrain from
amative indulgence.

Great numbers of women can easily refrain, for they
have no desire, and no enjoyment.   Either they are
born so, or have lost the power of pleasure by early
abuse or excess, or by frequent child-birth, or abortions and miscarriages.   In some way, they do not
possess, or they lose all sensibility.   But with many
women, also, it is voluntary.   While they submit to
the demands of their husbands, they can withhold any
participation.   They may become pregnant, all the
same.   Many women have families of children without

the least enjoyment of the sexual embrace. Women are sometimes deeply injured in their nervous systems by the efforts of their husbands to make them participate in, and so heighten, their enjoyments.

Certain kinds of food and drinks stimulate the amative propensity and its organism. "Oysters and eggs are amatory food," which is also true of game, fish, and of animal food generally; whose effect is much increased by salt, pepper, and spices. Coffee and chocolate and all rich wines have the same effect. Strong coffee is one of the most active of amatory stimulants. Alcohol does not so much stimulate lust, as dull the sense of caution, and the scruples that restrain men and women from enjoyment. The woman who drinks with her lover, is in his power.

There are drugs which quiet the amative feeling. This sedative influence is attributed to tobacco; and *satyriasis* in men, and *furor uterinus* in women— manias of unbridled lust—are treated with doses of the carbonates of sodium and potassium. A full diet provokes to lust; so does idleness of mind or body. The vital force must act in some direction; and if we would not have it expended on alimentiveness and amativeness, we must direct it to other and nobler uses. Perfect temperance, and even abstinence, or a pure, bland, simple, and very spare diet—bread, fruit, and cooling vegetables for food, and water for drink, with the love and desire of purity, and a varied activity of body and mind, are the best remedies. He who bathes daily, takes much active exercise, abstains from stimulants, lives on simple fare, does not eat after four o'clock, and sleeps on a hard bed with a light covering, will have little trouble from a disordered amativeness.

It is evident to every observer of human nature that the influence of sex runs through the whole mental and moral character. Men differ from women as much in brain as in body. They have certain organs relatively larger, and others relatively smaller, than women. The moral organs correspond intimately with all physical differences.

If we could compare the most masculine woman with the most feminine man, there would still be a wide difference. But this wide difference does not prove that woman was intended to be the slave, the tool, and the victim of man, as she is and has been. In making her such, man wrongs his own nature as much as he wrongs hers, and he wrongs the whole human race. If man would follow his own pure instincts, woman would have nothing to complain of and nothing to desire. By the rights of her love, by the power of her beauty, by the strength and tenderness of her passional nature, she would be acknowledged as the queen of the social universe; while man would reign in the sphere of intellect and material achievement.

It cannot be necessary in a Christian country to speak of those unnatural sexual crimes which shock society, and are sometimes punished by the laws. The sin of Sodom is found to some extent in the army, the navy, and in prisons, and is not unknown in the Metropolis. We read in the papers brief mention of prosecutions for other unnatural crimes. Incest, alas, is so common among the crowded populations of the very ignorant and very poor, that it is seldom punished. The marriages of near relations are also far too frequent; for there can be no doubt of their bad effect upon the bodily and mental organisation of their offspring. In a true society there would be no marriages of interest or consanguinity. The law of love is like that of magnetism—the attraction of opposites.

CHAPTER X.

EVOLUTION OF THE FŒTUS.

THE ovum once impregnated, Nature, by which I mean the informing soul that presides over the whole organic system, and gives intelligent guidance to every part, carries forward its development, as nearly as can be observed, in the following order:

The ovum is, from the first, enveloped in two membranes, the outer of which is called the chorion, the inner the amnion. Within lies the principle of life, the germ of the complex being. The ova of all the higher animals are alike at this period, and one cannot be distinguished from another. The amnion, or inner membrane, secretes upon its inner surface the liquid in which the fœtus is suspended during the whole period of gestation. The chorion, or outer covering, on the other hand, acts outwardly, throwing out villi, which, gathered at one point, at a certain period unite with vessels on the inner surface of the uterus, and form the placenta, or afterbirth, by which the fœtus is nourished from the blood of the mother.

The central germinal point of the egg, and its two coverings, form the three parts of a regular cell formation—cell, nucleus, and nucleolus.

While the ovum is gradually passing down the fallopian tube, propelled by the action of its ciliary bodies, a journey which lasts from eight to fourteen days, and in the course of which it is liable to impregnation, the uterus is preparing for its reception. A delicate secretion is poured out over its whole internal surface, which is organised into a membrane called the decidua, so that when the ovum arrives at the lower end of its fallopian tube, or one of the horns of the uterus, this decidua bars its entrance. But as the ovum is pushed forward, the membrane gives way, and is folded around the ovum, so as to make a double covering. The outer portion is called the decidua vera, or true membrane; the inner, the decidua reflexa, or folded membrane.

We have the ovum now protected by no less than four membranes—two proper to itself, the amnion and chorion, and the two formed by the folded decidua of the uterus.

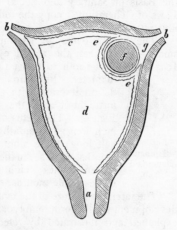

Fig. 33.—Ovum Entering the Uterus.*

During its passage down the fallopian tube, the entire ovum is so small that it is with great difficulty it can be found by the closest inspection and the aid of a powerful microscope. When found, however, and subjected to a high magnifying power, it exhibits the same phenomena as is displayed in the incubation of any other egg. There is the yolk, the germinal spot, which gradually expands, and the formation, first of blood, and an external circulation,

* Plan of the uterus at the moment when the ovum, *f*, sur-rounded by its chorion, *g*, is entering its cavity, and pushing the decidua vera before it to form the decidua reflexa. *a.* Neck c the uterus. *b, b.* Entrance to the fallopian tubes. *c,* Decidua vera, covering the walls of the uterus at every point. *d,* Cavity of the uterus.

and then of the rudimental organs; but these latter changes take place in the uterus.

From my more recent work, " HUMAN PHYSIOLOGY the Basis of Sanitary and Social Science," Part IV., Laws of Generation, I copy the following passage and illustrations :—

"The human ovum, at its impregnation, is very small—smaller than the naked eye can distinguish. It is from the 1-120th to the 1-140th of an inch in

diameter. But from the moment of fecundation it grows with great energy. In a fortnight it is of the size represented in Fig. 34. The fœtus of one month is an inch long; two months, two inches and a half long; three months, five inches; five months, six or seven inches; seven months, eleven inches; eight months, fourteen inches; nine months, eighteen inches.

Fig. 34.
Human
Ovum laid
open.

"The interior structure of the ovum, and the gradual development of the germ, embryo, and fœtus, are best explained and illustrated by reference to the larger

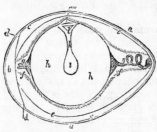

eggs of fishes and birds. The hen's egg may be taken as a model, and when a hen is setting, or, more humanely, when eggs are being hatched by artificial heat, if one be broken every second or third day, the whole development may be watched with great facility.

Fig. 35.—Ideal Section of a Hen's
Egg.*

---

* The egg of the fowl is the type of all ova, and from its large size is easy to study. *a, a.* Shell. *b.* Space filled with air to supply oxygen. *c.* Membrane of the shell, which, at *d, d,* splits

Nature, it will be seen, has prepared everything, forgotten nothing, and goes on in the formation of a new being, insect, bird, or man, with the same wisdom and power that creates a universe.

"The first step in development in the yolk of the egg must be the vitalisation of its matter—further vitalisation, I should say, for it is already alive—an organised existence. But the entrance of the masculine element

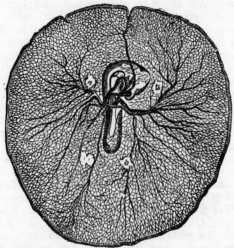

Fig. 36.—Chicken's Egg, Third Day of Incubation.

into two layers. *e, e.* Limits of the second and thicker albumen. *f.* Limits of the third and thickest albumen, the white being in three layers. *g, g.* Chalazæ, or ropes of twisted fibres from the yolk, which hold it in its place. *h.* Yolk. *i.* Central cavity in the yolk, from which a duct, *k,* leads to the cicatricula, or tread. *l.* Cumulus proligerous, or germinal cumulus. *m.* Germ, or blastos. The egg is so formed that the yolk floats high in the white, and the germ is always uppermost.

—or its union with the feminine element, whatever they may be—gives a new and very intense life. There is a diffusion, perhaps a rapid spreading growth of fibres of the nerves of organic life. Under their influence cells are formed of matter already fitted for such structures. These cells undergo rapid transformations, and become the blood, muscle, bone, all the tissues of the young animal. In the egg, these cells are seen to become more opaque in some parts, more transparent in others; they divide and subdivide, until the yolk forms what is called a mulberry mass. A germ gathers upon the surface, and separates into three layers. In the eggs of fishes, which are so transparent as to be easily watched through the process of development, may be seen an upper or nervous layer, in which are formed the organs of animal life—bones, muscles, brain and nerves, etc. The lower layer gives origin to the organs of vegetative life—the abdominal viscera, intestines, or alimentary system; the intermediate layer produces the heart, arteries, veins, etc., of the system of circulation.

"At a very early period, the general form of the insect or animal is manifested. In insects and crustaceans, the germ is divided into sections. In the germs of vertebrate animals, there is seen the rudiments of a spinal canal, which, when formed, is filled with a fluid, from which is formed the brain and spinal cord. The embryo rests upon the yolk, and covers it like a cap, vertebrates enclosing it by the edges uniting at the navel.

"In fishes, whose embryonic development has been carefully observed by Professor Agassiz, the first lines of the embryo appear on the tenth day—a canal, which becomes a tube—the spine, and an enlargement at one end, the rudimentary head, in which may soon be seen a division of the brain for the organs of sight, hearing, and smell; and soon after the rudiments of

eye and ear are apparent.   About the seventeenth
day the heart is seen as a simple cavity, and, as soon
as it is closed, there are regular contractions and a
movement of blood corpuscles.   On the thirtieth day
there is a regular circulation of blood; the tail gets
free, and moves in violent jerks, and the head is soon
liberated.   The fish has a brain, an intestine, a pulsating heart, and a limited amount of spontaneous
motion; but its form is not clearly defined.   By the
fortieth day, the shape of the fish is evident, the
remains of the yolk hang in a bag to its belly, but
it soon becomes absorbed, and then the fish is obliged
to seek its own food, having exhausted its embryonic
provision.

"The condition of the fish about the thirtieth day is
shown in the embryo of the fowl as early as the eighth
day — Fig. 37, where the
head forms more than half
the animal, and the eye is
out of all proportion to the
head.   The yolk is being
absorbed through a mem-
brane and vessels, which
unite to form the umbilicus,
the yolk of the egg being to
the embryo-chicken what
the placenta and blood of
the mother are to the human
fœtus."

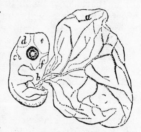

Fig. 37. —Embryo Fowl
of Eight Days.*

In the uterus, the growth of the new being is rapid.
Still, in the human subject, up to the seventh day,
nothing is visible to the naked eye.   On the tenth

* A further advanced embryo, with an apparatus of nutrition,
called the allantois, *a*, with the umbilical vessels, *b*, branching
over it.   *c*. The external ear.   *d*. Cerebellum.   *f*. Hemispheres.
The eye is very large, and far advanced; the mouth begins to
take the shape of a bill, and the legs and wings are sprouting.

day, there may be perceived a semi-transparent, grayish flake. On the twelfth there is a vesicle, nearly of the size of a pea, filled with fluid, in the middle of which swims an opaque spot, presenting the first appearance of an embryo, which may be clearly seen as an oblong or curved body, according as it is viewed, and plainly visible to the naked eye on the fourteenth day. The entire weight of the embryo and its two investing membranes, waters, etc., is now about one grain.

The increase from the first is astonishingly rapid, when we consider its original minuteness. On the twenty-first day the embryo resembles an ant, or a lettuce-seed;

Fig. 38.—Mammal Ovum.*

its length is four or five lines, and it weighs three or four grains. Many of its parts now begin to show themselves, especially the cartilaginous beginnings of the bones of the spinal column, the heart, brain, etc.

On the thirteenth day the embryo is as large as a horse-fly, and resembles a worm bent together. There are as yet no limbs, and the head is larger than the rest of the body. When stretched out, the embryo is nearly half an inch long.

In the seventh week bone begins to form in the lower jaw and clavicle. Narrow streaks on each side of the vertebral column show the beginning of the ribs; the heart is perfecting its form; the brain enlarged, and the eye and ear growing more perfect, and the limbs sprouting from the body. The lungs are mere sacs, about one line in length, and the trachea is a delicate thread, but the liver is very large. The

---

* Fig. 38 gives a view of the ovum of a bitch, twenty-three days from the last access of the male. The chorion has already shot forth little villi, which, however, are wanting at either end of the ovum, and also over the place where the embryo is situated. This engraving represents its object of the natural size.

anus is still imperforate. In the seventh week are formed the renal capsules and kidneys, and the sexual organs are speedily evolved, but the sex of the fœtus

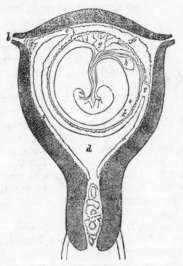

Fig. 39.—Fœtus in Utero.*

is not determined until some time after. The embryo is now nine lines, or three-fourths of an inch, in length.

---

* Sectional view of the uterus with the ovum; the cervix uteri is plugged up with a gelatinous mass, *a*. The decidua vera, *c*, sends a process, *c2*, into the right fallopian tube; the cavity of the uterus is almost completely occupied by the ovum. *e, e.* Points of reflection of the decidua reflexa. *f.* Decidua serotina. *g.* Allantois. *h.* Umbilical vesicle, with its pedicle in the umbilical cord. *i.* Amnion. *k.* Chorion; between the two, the space for the albumen.

In the eighth week the embryo is an inch long, weighs a drachm, and begins to show the division of fingers and toes.

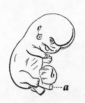

Fig. 40.
Human Embryo.

At from sixty to seventy days, the development is rapid, and all the parts are in the course of progressive formation. The eyes enlarge, the lids are visible, the nose grows prominent, the mouth enlarges, the external ear is formed, the brain is soft and pulpy, the neck well defined, and the heart fully developed. At three months, the eyelids are distinct, but shut, the lips are drawn together, the organs of generation very prominent in both sexes, both penis and clitoris being remarkably elongated. The heart beats with force, the larger vessels carry red blood, the fingers and toes are well defined, muscles begin to be developed, and the fœtus is four or five inches in length, and weighs about two and a half ounces.

At four months, it has greatly expanded in all its parts. The abdominal muscles are formed, and the intestines are no longer visible.

At five months, the lungs have increased, and are even susceptible of a slight dilatation. The skin is now in process of formation, the place of the nails is marked, and meconium gathers in the intestines, showing the action of excretory glands. Length, eight or ten inches; weight, fourteen or sixteen ounces.

At six months, a little down appears upon the head, the areolar tissue is abundant, and fat begins to be deposited. Length, nine to twelve inches; weight one pound.

At seven months, every part has increased in volume and perfection; the bony system is nearly complete. Length, twelve to fourteen inches; weight, two and a half to three pounds. This is reckoned as the epoch of viability, or the period in which the fœtus, if expelled from the uterus, is capable of independent existence.

From this period up to nine months, there is a mere increase of size and action. The red blood circulates in the capillaries, and the skin performs the function of perspiration. Length, eighteen to twenty-two inches; weight, from five to eight pounds.

There are cases in which an ill-nurtured fœtus, at its full period, does not weigh more than two or three pounds; on the other hand, cases are not rare in which the weight is twelve or fifteen pounds.

During the first weeks of the evolution of the embryo in the uterus, it is nourished, as the young chicken is, by the yolk of the egg. But soon the villi of the chorion gather into a compact mass, and become adherent to some portion of the uterus. There is formed thus a placenta, made of two portions, the maternal side, toward the walls of the uterus, and the fœtal, in which the vessels unite into two arteries and one vein, which, with their envelopments, form the umbilical cord, and communicate with the fœtal heart. By this means, at every pulsation of the heart, blood

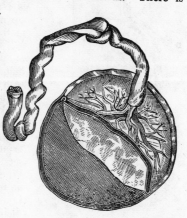

Fig. 41.—The Placenta and Umbilical Cord.

is sent through the two umbilical arteries to the placenta. Here the vessels branch out into capillaries, which mingle with those of the maternal placenta, communicating with the uterus. Through the membranous coats of these vessels, the blood of the foetus is nourished and purified. It receives nutritious matter and oxygen; it gives out carbonic acid. The placenta answers for the foetus then, the double purpose of stomach and lungs. The foetus has its own individual circulation and life; but all its nutriment, from the time this connection is formed, until it is severed at birth, comes from the mother.

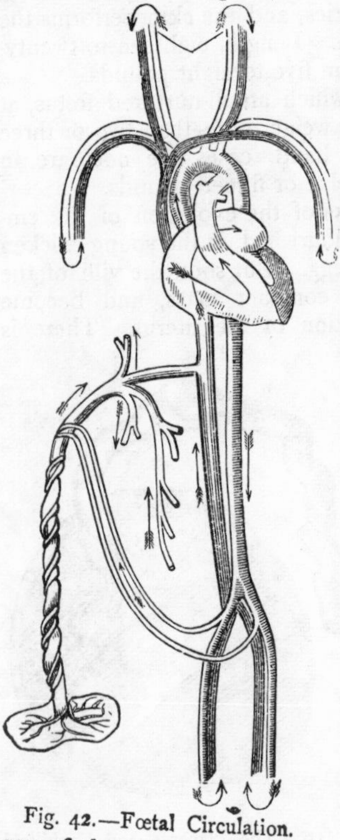

The regular period of pregnancy in the human female ends with the tenth lunar month, or fortieth week. Physiologists have asked why the process necessary to expulsion should be set up at this period. When they have given an intelligible explanation of any vital periodicity whatever, they may of this. Time is one of the elements of the universe, whether marked

Fig. 42.—Foetal Circulation.

by the beatings of the heart, and the movements of respiration, or the cycles of the stars, which require millions of millions of years for their completion. Regularities of action, and consequent accuracy of periods, are inherent qualities of the intelligent soul, animal or organic. It is the organic soul that presides over the development of the fœtus, and fixes the time for its expulsion. But this intelligent soul is not a machine. It has the power, for good reasons, to bring on the process of labour earlier, or postpone it to a later period.

The normal period of pregnancy is forty weeks, or nine months, reckoning from the last menstrual period. But as some persons have a quicker pulse than others, so, in some, the vital processes may be more rapid. There are also diseased irregularities which vary the time. Even domestic animals vary weeks in their periods. A gestation, even in a tolerably healthy woman, may be prolonged two or three weeks, and, in disease, still further. On the other hand, it may come on prematurely.

There have been cases where a fœtus of six months has been born, and lived; but seven months is generally considered the period of viability. At this time, even where miscarriages are artificially produced, it is said that two children out of three live. A reasonable man may be satisfied of the legitimacy of his child, if he has not been absent from its mother more than ten months at the period of its birth; and if he can count eight months from his first connection to the birth of a full-grown infant, he has no reason to be dissatisfied. Seven months children are said to occur oftenest in a first pregnancy.

There is no probability, I might say, possibility, that when the uterus is occupied by one fœtus, and all avenues to the ovaries are blocked up, another later conception can take place. But there is no reason wny a woman may not have twins by two fathers, who have connection with her at nearly the same time; and there are several cases in which twins have been born, one white and the other mulatto, or mulatto and black, in which the mother avowed that such a state of facts existed. In the same way, a litter of pups may be sired by several males, each pup bearing a resemblance to its particular father.

CHAPTER XI.

OF PREGNANCY.

I HAVE something to say now of the condition of the mother, and of her relation to her offspring during the interesting period of gestation. And first, how she may know when conception has taken place. A woman has reason to believe herself pregnant when several circumstances combine to render it probable.

1. If she has had sexual connection at the proper period; that is within five days before or ten days after the monthly period.

2. If, after sexual connection, the periodical discharge does not again occur.

3. If she have nausea in the morning, with unaccustomed antipathies or likings for persons and things.

4. If she have sharp pains in her breasts and a dark areola around the nipple, with pimples.

5. If she have a difficulty in restraining her urine.

6. If, after a short time, there is a gradual enlargement of the abdomen, becoming rapid and evident at the third or fourth month.

7. If she feel the motions of the child at and after this period.

Not one of these signs is certain; yet, where they all exist, there is a pretty strong probability. Thus, a woman may have sexual intercourse for years without conception; the menstrual function may cease from numerous derangements of the system; hysteria, or any ovarian irritation, may occasion strange mental peculiarities, antipathies, or longings; pains in the breast and areola may arise from similar causes; there may be irritation of the neck of the bladder, from falling or other displacements of the uterus; the abdomen may enlarge from tumor, dropsy, or even obstructed menstruation; and the motions of a child are often simulated by wind in the bowels and spasmodic affections.

There are signs, however, which are more certain, with a careful professional examination. After the third month it is possible to hear the beating of the foetal heart, by placing the ear, or a stethoscope, upon the mother's abdomen; possible to hear the *souffle* of the blood in the placenta; and to feel the weight of the foetus upon the point of the finger, properly applied at its lowest part, within the vagina. The first is a certain sound; the second may be confounded with other vascular action; and in the third case a tumor in the uterus may not be distinguishable from a foetus. An old writer, in speaking of the caution to be used in doubtful cases, says you must never give a decided opinion, until you have the child's head in your hand.

At a certain period of foetal growth, there occurs a rapid increase, a rising of the uterus in the abdomen, and muscular motion in the foetus; and this period is called the quickening. There is a notion that the foetus acquires a vitality or personality at this period, and that it is a greater crime to procure an abortion after than before it. There is not the slightest physiological ground for such an idea. The principle of life is there from the first. The act is essentially the same, at whatever period it is performed; or, if there is any difference in criminality, it is a gradual increase, according to the period, from the first day to the last.

The ovum belongs to the mother—she alone has a right to decide whether it shall be impregnated. That decision must be based upon her mental and physical condition, her desire for offspring, her ability to take proper care of it, and her social relations. But when a woman has united with a man in the creative act, the life of the being so formed is sacred. From the moment of conception it is a human life with all its possibilities, temporal and eternal.

There may be circumstances which justify the procurement of abortion, or the untimely expulsion of the embryo, or fœtus; such as a degree of deformity that prevents delivery. In such a case no medical man would hesitate to sacrifice the fœtus, to protect the life of the mother. This is as far, perhaps, as his responsibility extends. If a woman destroys her unborn offspring, to save what is more than life to her, and to avoid what is to many worse than death, we may pity her; but her action cannot be justified. It is an act of murder; a crime against nature.

But it is a very common crime among tribes of savages, and in the highest civilisation. In America, and to some extent probably in every country in Europe, there are persons, physicians and others, who make a living—fortunes in some instances—by giving drugs, or performing operations to procure abortions, not only on girls, to save them from disgrace, but upon married women, to relieve them from the inconveniences of childbearing.

There are various modes of procuring abortion; and as this is, in all cases, a violent and unnatural process, it is always attended with a degree of danger, chiefly from a liability to uterine hemorrhage, or flooding.

The most common mode of procuring abortion is by sexual intercourse during pregnancy. Every woman who permits it, does it with this risk. When a woman is weak in constitution, or strongly amative; when a man is violent in his manifestations, or the womb is low, there is always the liability to procure the expulsion of the fœtus. All amative excitement on the part of the female perils the existence, as it injures the proper growth, and injuriously affects the character of the child. The excited uterus expels the embryo, and in thousands of cases this goes on, year after year, and people wonder they have no children. Women who have neither passion nor pleasure are less liable to abortion from this cause than others; but if procuring abortion be a crime, is it less so when done in this mode, and without any proper motive?

Violent exercise of the body, or violent passions of the mind, tend to abortion and miscarriage. Women of weak constitutions should carefully avoid both.

Errors of diet, exhausting labours and cares, bring on abortions and miscarriages. They use up the stock of vitality, or the organic force which should go to the fœtus. It dies, and is expelled. So perish thousands of unborn infants; and as care and poverty increase in our great cities, so increase the number of still-born children.

The use of drugs and the lancet is a prolific cause. Whatever depresses or deranges the vital functions may be a cause of abortion. Blood-letting and drug poisoning do both. There is no doubt that thousands of infant germs are poisoned in the uterus by allopathic medication, while still more are born diseased from the same cause. The doctor poisons the blood of the mother, and from this the blood of the child draws its nourishment.

When abortion is wilfully procured, it is by one of two methods—drug poisoning or a surgical opera-

tion. In the former the mother is poisoned, sometimes fatally, in the effort to expel the child. The
surgical method, that of rupturing the membranes, is
the simplest method, but not unattended with danger.
The most recent plan is to introduce a slender bougie
into the uterus and let it remain until it induces contractions.

In a proper social condition, I see no reason why
any woman should ever desire to procure an abortion.
In the prevalent unnatural conditions of society, and
the diseased state of women, morally and physically,
it has become a custom of shocking frequency.

The direct physical influence of the father upon the
child ceases with the act of impregnation. All after
influence must be through the mother, or of an aromal,
or what is termed a magnetic character. If the woman,
in this interesting period of her life, is folded day and
night in the arms of love, and lives in an atmosphere
of tender care, she receives strength every hour, and
the child may be directly a partaker of the loving
father's life. But there is no question of the influence
of the mother. If her blood is pure, the child is built
up in purity. If she has an abundant vitality, her
child drinks from a full fountain. Every thing that
disorders the mother affects the child. If ever all
the laws of health are strictly obeyed, it should be
during gestation.

An impression upon the mother, of any kind, acts
upon the child. Children are born happy or miserable, according to the state of their mothers during
pregnancy, just as they are born healthy or diseased.
Particular talents, tendencies, tastes, idiosyncrasies, and
affections of every kind, are impressed upon them, and
govern their future lives. The mother of Napoleon,
while carrying him, accompanied her husband in a
military campaign. The most extraordinary peculiarities are inflicted upon children by some temporary

condition of the mother; and there is abundant proof that this may extend to the body as well as the mind. The facts of this character have been denied by mere theorists, because they cannot account for them. Alas! for what can they account?

Such observations as I have been able to make, induce me to think that the sex of a child is determined by the relative vigour of the parents. The father, from maturity, force of will, or superior strength of the procreative function, may give the masculine development; or the mother, from similar causes, may give the feminine. Where men of mature age cohabit with women much younger, there is an excess of males; but in countries where the customs of polygamy prevail, and a man's vital force is expended on several women, there will be more daughters than sons born to him; so that polygamy perpetuates itself. Where monogamic relations prevail, the sexes are born in nearly equal numbers.

Pregnant women are sometimes affected with the most extraordinary longings, and there is a prevailing impression that they must have what they long for, however absurd or hurtful. A woman has longed for a quart of brandy a day, and drank it. Women eat the most nauseous and indigestible substances. These are states of disease, and should be treated as such. If the article longed for is harmless, as some particular fruit, it should be procured, if possible; but no woman should be allowed to take arsenic because she longs for it, nor anything else that is positively and necessarily hurtful. The pregnant woman should live on the most simple diet, refraining at this time, above all others, from every thing of a mischievous or doubtful nature; bathing regularly, taking exercise, and living in the most exact obedience to the laws of life. Doing this, she will escape hysterical and insane longings, or be able to overcome them, with great benefit to herself, and without mischief to her child.

All observation shows that not only are the striking characteristics of races transmitted, for thousands of years, as with the negroes, the Chinese, the Jews, etc., but that the qualities and peculiarities of every in dividual are in like manner transmissible. It is proven also that any faculty exercised during pregnancy by the mother, is strengthened in the child. Thus any mental or moral faculty of the mother may be made striking and active in the child, by being used during pregnancy; and in this way every mother has in her charge, in a great measure, not only the physical, but the mental and moral character of her offspring.

And it is for these reasons that every child should be a child of love, a child of health, and all generous activities; a child of competence, and freedom from care and the miseries of poverty; a child of beauty, begotten and developed amid beautiful things and beautiful thoughts; a child of frank, honest sincerity. If we would improve our race, we must give to the mothers of our race all the conditions of improvement and happiness.

The whole process of gestation, it should be remembered, is a natural process, and every part of it should be naturally performed, from the beautiful act of impregnation, sanctified by the holy passion of love, and accompanied with the most exquisite of all sensual delights, to the grand act of the expulsion of the fœtus, and its entrance upon independent life. And this whole process, when accomplished naturally, is one of delight, and not by any means one of disease and pain. Even the process of childbirth, with such a degree of health and strength as may be gained by the water-cure, and a physiological regimen, is rendered speedy, and almost entirely painless.

The pain of any organic action is caused by disease. Where there is no disease, there can be no pain. There is no reason why the contractions of the uterus may not be as painless as those of the bladder; and where this organ is in perfect health, they are so. All that a woman wants to secure a painless labour is perfect health; and her labours will be free from pain, and free from danger, just in proportion as she becomes a healthy being.

I have known many cases in which women who have had long, painful, and perilous labours, have by pure diet, exercise, bathing, and other health conditions, come into such a state of vigour as to pass through this trying period with no danger and very little suffering.

During the nine months of pregnancy, in which the happy expectant mother carries the growing babe in her womb, her person should be sacred, her passions calm, her mind serene and full of peace and hope and happiness. No work should weary her, no anxiety disturb her, no lust excite or torment her. She should have daily moderate exercise in the open air, walking or driving; plenty of fresh, pure air by night and by day; daily bathing in cold water, with the frequent use of the sitz bath, the wet bandage, and, if possible, the fountain bath, or rising douche or spray; and also of the vaginal syringe, when there is such need, as will be pointed out in further chapters. Her diet should be moderate, simple, pure, and perfectly healthful; consisting chiefly of brown bread and its equivalents, fruit, milk, vegetables, with little, if any, flesh meat. No heating or exciting condiments, and no tea, coffee, or alcoholic stimulants. Her whole life, in short, should be as natural and therefore as healthful as she can make it. And in her body, and mind, and soul, she should be just what she would wish her unborn child to be in all its future life; for its health and happiness depend in a great measure on the state of the mother during this important period.

CHAPTER XII.

SYMPTOMS OF HEALTH.

MEDICAL books are filled with descriptions, symptoms, and causes of disease. I wish to give a clear description, enumerate the symptoms, and guide my reader to a knowledge of the conditions of health.

Doctors have not been, as a rule, required to keep people in health, but to cure their diseases. It is very seldom that a man sends for a physician and says to him, "We are all, thank God, in pretty good health, and I want you to give us such directions as will keep us so." People wait until they are ill, and then send for the doctor to cure them. Therefore, it is not the interest of doctors to study health, but disease; it is not their interest to preserve the health of the public —their living depends upon the contrary condition. If doctors were paid in proportion to the health of the community, and their incomes were diminished by every epidemic, and every case of disease, we should stand in less need of sanitary legislation.

Physicians are interested in disease, as soldiers are in war and lawyers in quarrels. If we had professional peace-makers between individuals and nations, and professional health-makers, well paid for their successful efforts—paid and honoured in proportion to their success—it might be different. As it is, it is not for the interest of any physician that health should prevail in communities, that any individual should remain free from sickness, or that he should recover rapidly. Every day the cure is expedited, takes money out of his pocket, and bread out of the mouths of his family.

HEALTH is, to every organised being, the condition

of perfect development; to every sentient being the condition of happiness.

HEALTH, in a human being, is the perfection of bodily organisation, intellectual energy, and moral power.

HEALTH is the fullest expression of all the faculties and passions of man, acting together in perfect harmony.

HEALTH is entire freedom from pain of body, and discordance of mind.

HEALTH is beauty, energy, purity, holiness, happiness.

HEALTH is that condition in which man is the highest known expression of the power and goodness of his Maker.

When a man is perfect in his own nature, body and soul, perfect in their harmonious adaptations and action, and living in perfect harmony with nature, with his fellow-man, and with God, he may be said to be in a state of HEALTH.

If the organs of the body are all fully developed and in full action, they must necessarily be in harmony; and when a man is in harmony in himself, he is of necessity in harmony with all men, all nature, and with the Source of all things.

It is therefore necessary that every minute organ of the body, every faculty of the mind, every power of the soul should be fully formed and active—all balancing and harmonising each other; that man should act out all the fulness of his nature, and woman all the glorious beauty of her character, in perfect freedom, and in full enjoyment, to make up the integral condition of HEALTH.

BEAUTY is the first sign of health. Health gives development; and harmonious development is beauty. Every vegetable and every animal is beautiful, according to its own type of beauty, when it is most perfectly

developed. And in man or woman, the exact development of every part, and that which enables it to best
perform its function, is the highest possible beauty. The
handsomest possible head is the one which has the
most perfect phrenological developments. The most
beautiful eye, ear, or nose, are those best adapted to
seeing, hearing, and smelling. The loveliest mouth
has the best shaped lips and most perfect teeth. The
most delicious bosom is the one best fitted for its
natural office. The finest limbs are those with the
best muscular development. In a word, there is no
part of the human figure where the best condition for
use is not, at the same time, the condition of the highest
beauty, and both together are synonymous with health.
Consequently, every deformity, every ugliness, every
departure from the standard of the highest beauty of
its kind, is a consequence and symptom of disease.

O ye, who love beauty, and who desire it for your-
selves, for your offspring, and for the race, learn that
the single way to attain it is by the practice of the laws
of health. Be good, and you shall be beautiful as well
as happy. Let no man who has a love for nature and
a reverence for God undervalue beauty. It is to be
sought, admired, loved and worshipped.

Another symptom of health is ACTIVITY. Every
healthy nerve has a desire to use its power ; every
healthy muscle wishes to contract ; every healthy faculty wishes to find exercise and consequent enjoyment.
This rule extends to the organic, as well as the animal
system. In health the secretions are active, and so
are the excretions; there is a sharp appetite, quick
digestion, a full circulation, an earnest respiration, and
everywhere an active nutrition. Body and mind are
active. All the passions spring into spontaneous activities, alternating with each other, and all contributing
to that great variety of action and sensation which
constitute the complex phenomenon of Life.

Indolence, on the other hand, is a consequence and a sign of disease. A torpid organ is a diseased organ. A lazy man is a sick man. Give him health, and his laziness will vanish. Every well man is a busy man. There is no tendency to indolence in a healthy person. The real tendency is to high activities; and the healthier the world grows, the more varied and active will be its industry.

STRENGTH, or energy, is a sign of health; though a kind of discordant strength, or spasmodic energy, may be a mark of disease. But steady power comes from integrity of constitution. There must be good brain, good nervous fluid, and good muscular fibre, before we can have real strength, and true persistent energy of character and action. These must come from a deep vitality. Men of strong desires, strong passions, strong wills, have strong lives; and a strong life is generally a long and healthy one.

Weakness—mental, or passional, or physical—is a sign of disease, as it is a consequence. It is want of development, or exhaustion, or hereditary taint, or acquired morbid condition, or all together, one producing the other. If we blame the weak, the vascillating, the craving, the spiritless, nerveless, hopeless, purposeless, we must blame them only for what has brought them to this condition. It is a condition of disease, which, if possible, we must cure.

HAPPINESS is a sign of health, and withouth health a full enjoyment of life cannot exist. A condition of happiness is said to be "a sound mind in a sound body." This is a simple description of a healthy condition. Happiness is the end or final cause of all sentient life. There is no other conceivable reason for the creation of any being. Happiness is, therefore, the positive and necessary result of every true life, as misery is the inevitable, because equally necessary, result of a false life. As health is the condition

L

of a true life, the result and sign of health is happiness.

Hence all unhappiness of every kind, all pain, grief,
regret, jealousy, discontent, anxiety, is the result of
disease, bodily or mental, in ourselves or others. Sorrow seems to me just as much the effect of a disease
as pain. One is the outcry of a sick organism, the
other of a wounded spirit. We feel sorrow by sympathy with others; and there are many persons of
sensitive organisations who feel bodily pain the same
way. The way to be happy is to be healthy; and
when health is universal, there is no conceivable reason why there should be any unhappiness. There is
no happiness without a corresponding degree of health,
and no health without a corresponding degree of happiness.

CHAPTER XIII.

THE CONDITIONS OF HEALTH.

As health is the simple, natural state of man, when his
whole development and life are in accordance with the
laws of his being, the CONDITIONS OF HEALTH are
entirely based on the science of physiology or anthropology.

What I prefer to call the conditions of health include
the whole science of hygiene, and these conditions are
the basis of the laws of life. Without a full observance
of them, no human being can have health, which includes in itself beauty, activity, energy, happiness.
Without a full observance of them, humanity is liable
to ugliness, deformity, pains, and every complication of
misery, all of which are included in the idea of disease

These conditions of health cannot be observed, if they are not known. We have so neglected a knowledge of ourselves, so perverted ourselves, so far gone astray from nature, that a pure, simple, natural life is almost unknown to us. Our souls are perverted by unnatural beliefs, notions, and habits of thought, as our bodies are by absurd customs, fashions, and habits of action. There is a curious correspondence between our mental and bodily perversions. In both ways, we are out of harmony with nature, and at discordance in ourselves.

The first condition of health to every living thing is to be well begotten. The farmer who wishes good crops, selects his seed with care. He does not expect large, clean, sound wheat from small, smutty, shrivelled seed; healthy lambs from diseased sheep and rams; good cows and strong oxen from a poor, diminutive breed; nor a beautiful, fleet horse from an inferior stock. Man is also an animal, and subject to all the laws of hereditary descent which govern the propagation of other animals.

Diseased parents beget diseased children; and the reverse. Long-lived parents beget long-lived children; and *vice versa*. There are causes which operate upon the individual in both cases, to modify the effects of hereditary predisposition. A man, gifted with a good constitution from his ancestry, may destroy the principle of longevity in his offspring, though he may live to a good age himself. So a man may transmit to his children a vigorous life-principle, which he may afterwards undermine in himself by his own bad habits. He may die early, in spite of a good constitution; while his children, inheriting his healthy organisation, may be more fortunate in preserving it.

To be well begotten, one's parents must not only be of a good stock, and have inherited and developed a good organisation, but they must be actually living healthy lives, and observing the conditions of health. Any unhealthy condition of the father affects the seminal fluid. For this to be pure and strong and vital, the blood and the nervous power must be in the same condition, and so of the germs prepared by the mother. No unhappy man, no diseased man, no man whose nervous power is exhausted by labour or care; no man who poisons his blood, and disorders his nerves with stimulants and drugs, can possibly beget a healthy child. Every zoosperm prepared in the testes for the fecundation of the ovum is affected by every cause that affects the parent. There is no condition of body or mind, with which the germ of life may not be affected by either of the parents. The seeds of all follies, vices, and crimes are sown in the organism. The Bible truly says of men, that they had certain characters "from the mother's womb." Moral character, intellectual powers and tendencies, physical organisation, health or disease, happiness or misery, are impressed upon the infinitesimal germ, and the inconceivably minute zoosperm. The microscopic animalcule, shaped like an elongated tadpole, is, in reality, a blackguard, a liar, a thief, a scoundrel; or it is scrofulous, or syphilitic, or gouty; or it is idiotic, or insane : all these, if formed by a parent of whom these are actual qualities. And so it is of the germ prepared in the ovary of the mother. So the sins of parents are visited on their children to the third and fourth generation, and, where the causes continue, to the thirtieth and fortieth.

Father and mother, therefore, at the time of begetting, must be in all pure, and natural, and healthy conditions. If the parents love each other, the child will love its parents. But if a woman submits to be impregnated by a man whom she loathes and hates, that loathing and hatred will be impressed upon the child. It will show it in infancy, and it often lasts through life. Mr. O. S. Fowler gives an account of a man who had never been able, from his birth, to look at his father, from the impression made upon him by the mother, previous to and during pregnancy. For these reasons, if for no others, sexual commerce should never take place but in a most loving union of congenial souls. Two persons may have sworn eternal love upon a "stack of Bibles;" but if they do not love, they have no right to have children. Sexual union should never take place in sickness, or depression, or fatigue, nor under the influence of stimulants. Mr. Combe has given a case in which an idiot was the product of sexual union during a drunken frolic. The world is full of miserable wretches, the results of sexual commerce forced upon a loathing wife by a drunken husband.

And from this primary condition of health comes the law, that every woman, by her supreme right to herself, has the right to choose when she will have a child, and by whom. She is to carry it, to bear it, to nurse it, to educate it ; she is responsible to her child for its paternity and its development; and this respon- sibility carries with it the right of choice in all that affects it.

When men are once enlightened on this subject, none but inhuman wretches and monsters will deny these rights. We talk of the evils of slavery, and of the sub- mission of female slaves to their masters' lusts. Look at the slavery of women over the civilised world, and their submission to the lusts of *their* masters.

Nature is ever kind, and neglects nothing that can benefit her creatures. She exerts her power to pre- serve the race, even from these evils. What some doctors call the *vis medicatrix naturæ*—the healing power of nature, which tends constantly to growth and healthy development, which heals our wounds, and cures our diseases when we give it a chance, and it is possible to do so ; this power operates ever to purify, strengthen, and elevate. It does much to save the child from the diseases of the parent, and children are often better than we could expect. With all things in nature working together for good, we must not despair, but try to improve by culture and education. With good conditions, and surrounded by good influences, the faults and diseases of birth are gradually eradicated and cured, until scarcely a sign of them remains; and children, born ugly, diseased, and with unfortunate mental and moral tendencies, may come to be more beautiful, healthy, and good than seemed possible in their infancy.

The second condition of health is, that a child should be well born, or, more properly, well *borne.* The whole state of the mother, during the period of pregnancy, influences the being of the child. Her blood is its nutriment, and that blood must be pure. It is from her nervous system that it derives the elements of its own vitality. Its mental and moral organisation is influenced by hers, and even by her thoughts and feelings. Its muscular structure may be made strong by her taking proper exercise, or weakened by her indolence. Children are born with club feet, because mothers would take no exercise during pregnancy. Children are born with dyspepsia, or a tendency to colic, from the mother eating improper food at this period. The food of the mother has so much to do with the condition of the child, and with her power to bring it forth at the proper period without pain or danger, that few things are more important. Numerous experiments prove that a fruit diet, or one composed chiefly of fruit, is the best possible. Too much farinaceous food, especially wheat, promotes the premature hardening of the bones, diminishes the flexibility of the fœtus, and increases the difficulty of parturition. No well-informed human mother will live on the flesh of animals during either gestation or lactation. Flesh is not fit to make babies, nor milk to feed them. There is no condition of the mother, mental or physical, which may not have its influence upon the child. How careful, then, should every mother be to live in the best possible conditions during this period; and how careful should all around her be to make her life happy! There is no condition of health necessary to the mother, which is not also necessary to the child, for it partakes of all her life.

When we reflect upon the poverty, material and spiritual, that exists everywhere; upon the discord that enters into the lives of those who are most fortunate; upon the evil habits of living that surround us; and all the vices and miseries by which women are enveloped, and to which they are exposed, can we wonder that half the children born die before they are five years old; that thirty years is the average length of human life, and that, with so many, this brief space is filled with pain and misery? Pork, tea, coffee, tobacco, beer, whisky, crowded and filthy dwellings, bad air, uncleanly habits, and corresponding pursuits, feelings, and passions, are not the materials of which healthy babies are made. Such babies die, must die, and ought to die. They are not fit to live, and such a life, when it is prolonged, is a curse, and not a blessing.

The same law applies, during the period of nursing, to the mother or the nurse. Every mother should nurse her own child, unless it would be better off without it. A healthy hired nurse is better than a diseased mother; but the life and habits of the nurse must be under the same control as the mother's. Neither mother nor nurse, during lactation, should ever be exposed to sexual excitement. Amative indulgence diminishes the quantity of milk, and hurts its quality. And where this indulgence excites menstruation, and results in pregnancy, there is a double misfortune. The child at the breast and the child in

the womb are both defrauded. There is no doubt
that the milk of a healthy, well-behaved cow is better
for a child than that of a sickly or vicious mother
or nurse. The food, the air, exercise, the feelings,
employments, and the whole state of body and mind,
influence the quality of the milk. The milk of an
indolent mother will not give strength to the child.
Even cows kept up in stalls, give milk with much
butter and little of the flesh-forming principle, or case-
ine. All narcotics, all stimulants, all drug poisons,
all impurities in food, or air, or about the person, affect
the milk, and the child who feeds upon it. Many a
child is kept drunk on tea, or tobacco, or whisky. The
nurse drinks her porter or whisky, and the baby grows
stupid on milk-punch, drawn from her bosom. And
it is "such a good child!" "Nurses and sleeps all the
time." These are some of the ways in which children are poisoned, killed outright, or made stupid
drunkards. Tons of opium are given to the infants
of the poor, and they die by thousands in consequence; but there is not much mourning on account
of this murder of the innocents.

Natural food is a condition of health to every organised being. A plant finds its appropriate nourishment
in the air, or draws it from the earth. We do not
expect a vegetable to flourish in an uncongenial soil,
because it is the soil that furnishes a portion of the
matter necessary to its growth. It is the same with
animals. Every one, from the smallest to the largest,
is furnished with its appropriate food by bountiful
nature; and every animal but man eats in a natural
state the food that nature intended. The superiority
of man over all other animals, is proved by the extent
of his perversions. His greater capacity and freedom,
which enable him to do greater and nobler deeds,
enable him at the same time to do meaner and more
debasing ones.

Vegetables, by careful effort, may be made to grow in soils not specially adapted to nourish them, and in climates not best adapted to their production. So animals may be educated to live on unnatural diet, but this is never a condition of health. Thus cows upon a barren sea-shore learn to live on fish; a sheep has been taught to eat beefsteak and drink coffee; and a horse has acquired the filthy and disgraceful habit of chewing tobacco. But no sane man will say that these things are natural or healthy.

In the same way man learns to eat and love a great variety of unnatural and hurtful articles of food, such as are not adapted to his digestive organs, or the best nutrition of his system. He also learns to tolerate and love the most nauseous and detestable poisons, of which the wide-spread use of tobacco is a remarkable instance.

Man has, in accordance with the energy of his nature, and the versatility of his powers, a greater range of adaptiveness than any other animal. He can live in all climates, by the aid of artificial protection and heat, and he can live on a wide range of alimentary substances.

But all experience, all observation, and all science, prove that there are certain kinds of food especially adapted to the constitution of man—the same as in the case of other animals; and this food is best for health in its widest and most comprehensive meaning.

The essential nutriment of vegetables consists of four elements : oxygen, hydrogen, carbon, and nitrogen. These are all found in the atmosphere, in water, and the earth. The same elements are the most essential in animal organisations, but in animals they are obtained from the vegetable kingdom. Thus the vegetable kingdom rests upon the inorganic, and the animal upon the vegetable.

Though all animals live upon the products of the

vegetable kingdom, and though there is no particle of animal nutriment in the world which has not been elaborated by the vegetable kingdom from the inorganic, yet there are many animals who get this food at second-hand, and in various stages of impurity and disease.

Animals may be divided into three classes; the herbivorous, or vegetable-eating animals; the carnivorous, or flesh-eating; and the omnivorous, or those who feed upon both. Of vegetable-eating animals we have some who live upon the grasses and other coarse vegetation, such as the horse, cow, sheep, camel, elephant, etc., and others who live upon fruits, seeds, nuts, and roots. Of carnivorous beasts, we have some living on freshly killed animals, as the lion, tiger, panther, etc., while others feed on carrion, as the hyena, wolf, and many birds. The hog is the type of the omnivora. It eats everything—snakes, toads, carrion, excrement, as well as nuts, seed, fruits. Man, also, is held to belong to this class, and to be even more omnivorous than the hog himself. That he is so by perversion and habit, I shall not deny; but that he ever is so, in a natural and healthy state, all nature and all science deny.

Man has not the claws, nor the teeth, nor the digestive organs, nor the tastes or attractions of a carnivorous animal; neither has he those of a grass-eating animal. The teeth of a carnivorous animal are formed to tear, and rend, and cut in pieces. Man's teeth are made, the front for cutting, the back for mashing and grinding. Those of grass-eating animals are adapted to a peculiar cutting and grinding process, necessary for the comminution of

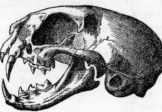

Fig. 43.—Skull of Carnivora.

coarse vegetable fibre. The digestive canal of the carnivora is shorter and simpler than that of man; that of the graminivora, or grass-eating tribes, is longer and more complicated.

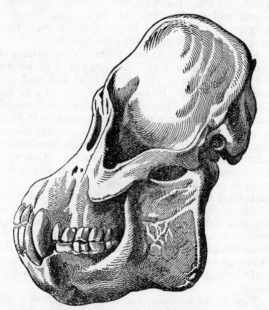

Fig. 44.—Skull of Orang Outang.

The animals whose teeth, digestive organs, and general physiology bear most resemblance to man, are of the class of frugivorous, or fruit-eating animals, at the head of which, and most resembling man, is the orang outang. This is a strong, active animal, growing to nearly the size of man, which lives on fruit, nuts, and roots.

The unperverted tastes of every animal point with unerring certainty to its natural diet. Wherever a decaying carcase taints the air, there will be found the foul creatures that feast on carrion—the hog, the hyena, the wolf, the crow, the buzzard, the vulture. Worms and insects finish the feast. The lion and tiger revel in the warm blood of the animals they have just slain, but turn away from carrion.

Now what are the natural tastes and attractions of man in respect to food. Reader, you shall be my judge. Let me take you by the hand, and lead you into this garden. It shall be, if you please, the Garden of Eden. Trees loaded with fruit are around you—vines bending with luscious grapes, beds filled with melons. Here are apples, pears, peaches, plums, nectarines, grapes, figs, oranges, bananas, strawberries, raspberries, and more than I can count. Here, also, are esculent roots, and nutritious seeds, fields of waving grain or golden maize, potatoes, beets, turnips. The air is filled with delicious odours; every object is full of beauty. Happy children are gathering fruit, or plucking flowers. All around are life and harmony, sweetness and purity, peace and happiness. The farm, the garden, the orchard, the vineyard, are full of beautiful associations, and not one object, if it properly belongs there, is offensive to the most refined taste.

Now, let us look upon another picture: A fœtid, sickening odour fills the air; shrieks and moans of agony salute you; the gutters run full of blood, but you must enter. A raging bull, with his frenzied eye glaring upon his murderers, is dragged up with horrid bellowings; a dull blow falls upon his skull, and the blood gushes from his throat. The strong, honest ox, who has toiled all his life for man, is murdered. The timid sheep, with painful bleatings, now feels the knife at its throat, and gasps away its innocent life. Calves, torn from their mothers, are hung up by their feet, their veins opened, and allowed to slowly bleed to death, that the veal may be white, drained of its blood, and tender, from the long death-agonies. Around you are the opened carcases of these, your fellow-creatures, and your friends—the floor is covered with their blood and entrails.

What sense is gratified by such a scene as this? Is it beautiful to the sight, pleasant to the ear, grateful to the smell, or does it awaken any calm or happy feeling?

If a man wished to take a walk with one he loved, would he go to a garden, or a slaughter-house? If he wished to send her a present, would it be a basket of fruit, or a string of sausages?

Man loves the vegetable world, and finds it full of beauty, and attraction, and gratification, because it is his. His nature is adapted to it; it is adapted to all his wants, and all his natural desires. It is not so with carnivorous and carrion animals. What care the lion, or tiger, or wolf, or hyena, or buzzard, for orange groves and fig trees, orchards and vines, fields of waving corn, or granaries with their rich winter stores?

Flesh-eating physiologists and physicians have contended for the necessity, if not the beauty, of eating animal food; but all experience, all science, and all philosophy, are arrayed against them. At this moment, and in all past time, nine-tenths of the whole human race have lived on a vegetable diet, either eating no flesh or making it the rare exception. The great mass of the labour of the world is done on a vegetable diet. In Japan, China, the whole East Indies, Persia, Turkey, all Europe, save the sea-coasts, all Africa, and Central America, flesh is seldom or never eaten by the poor, and over much of this territory, not even by the rich. The finest forms, the best teeth, the strongest muscles, the most active limbs in the world, are fed on a purely vegetable diet; while with regard to intellectual and moral development, it is a curious and interesting fact, that there can scarcely be mentioned a great philosopher or poet of ancient or modern times who has not given his testimony, either in his opinions or his practice, in favour of a vegetarian diet. Those who have any doubt on this subject, will do well to examine it fully.

In the Chemistry of Man, I have shown that not only are all the elements which are needed by the blood, and which enter into the human organism, found in vegetables; not only the ultimate elements, as carbon, oxygen, hydrogen, nitrogen, but the proximate elements, as albumen, fibrin, and fatty matter. And these elements are there in great abundance, and in great purity; in many cases in just the proportions in which they are needed, and free from all taint of disease. This is never the case with flesh used as food. The nutritive matters it contains are in wrong proportions, *and always mixed with the excrementitious matters passing out of the animal system, and often with the matter of disease;* for there are few animals fattened for slaughter, that are not diseased in the process, by being deprived of the conditions of health. Thus the flesh of the healthiest animal contains much waste and poisonous matter; while thousands of those eaten every day are one mass of disease. The details on this point are too disgusting to be written. We have only to read in the journals of the quantity of diseased and putrefying flesh condemned by the inspectors.

Fruit and the farinacea are the natural, and, therefore, the most healthy food for man. They are best fitted to sustain him in vigour of body and mind. They preserve him in health, and enable him to recover from disease. They contain all the elements he requires in the best proportions and in the best condition. A vegetarian diet is preëminently the diet of beauty, energy, activity, and enjoyment. It is the best at all ages, in all conditions, in all employments. It is the best for the labourer, as for the philosopher, the artist, the professional man, or the man of the world. On a vegetable diet, the skin grows clear, the cheeks rosy, the eyes bright, all senses acute, the wits sharp, the intellect vigorous, the feelings deep and pure, the digestion good, all functions regular, the passions under control, the temper calm, the intuitive perceptions quickened, and the whole being exalted into a new, more vigorous, and more beautiful life.

The diet most consistent with health, is one composed of the best ripe fruits, as strawberries, raspberries, whortleberries, peaches, pears, apples, grapes, melons, tomatoes, oranges, bananas, figs, dates; wheat, Indian corn, rice, oatmeal, rye, barley; peas, beans, lentils, asparagus, potatoes, beets, turnips, squash, cabbage, salsify, egg-plant, etc., etc. There is a vast variety, of which hundreds of the most exquisite dishes may be made. If we add two articles from the animal kingdom, procured without destruction of life, and which may generally be had in a state of tolerable purity, our list, if not complete, is sufficient for every reasonable desire—I mean milk and eggs. These furnish us with a concentrated aliment of agreeable flavour, and they mingle harmoniously with most vegetable substances.

The quantity of food, many persons say, who wish to gratify perverted tastes, is of more importance than quality. Each has its own special importance; but when a man eats food of the proper quality, he is not so apt to err in quantity, and his errors are not so mischievous. It is surely worse to eat too much of a bad thing, than too much of a good thing. A man is much more apt to kill himself with brandy than with potatoes. Vegetarian gluttons exist, doubtless, especially among those who have become diseased on other modes of diet; but they are not so common, I imagine, as among "riotous eaters of flesh."

The proper quantity of food for a mature healthy person should include about twelve ounces of nutriment per day. This is contained in rather less than one pound of farinaceous food, two pounds of potatoes, and what are called vegetables, and a still larger quantity of fruit.

Food may be taken, in early infancy, every two or three hours; and the frequency should be gradually diminished, until, at a year old, the child takes but three meals a day. For the adult, three meals, at intervals of six hours, seems a natural arrangement, though many persons advocate eating but two meals a day. The last meal, when three are eaten, should be lightest in quantity, and most easy of digestion.

The rules for eating are much like those of other functions. Hunger is nature's call for food, and supply should be governed by demand. We should never, when in health, eat but when we are hungry, nor drink but when we are thirsty. We should masticate thoroughly, which insures a proper insalivation. Even when the food is so soft as not to really require chewing to be swallowed, it ought to be well mixed with saliva. If the food be simple and pure, not too much sweetened or salted, nor prepared with exciting condiments, the sense of hunger is soon overcome, appetite is satisfied, and we feel that we have eaten enough.

We should never eat when fatigued, nor in any way exhausted; nor should we commence violent labour, bodily or mental, nor take a bath, immediately after eating. In the first case we prevent, in the second we interrupt, digestion. We want a large portion of our strength for digestion, and a good digestion gives us strength for every other purpose. Moderate exercise and pleasant mental excitement, as conversation or some amusement, rather favour the digestive process.

Salt, if necessary at all, which recent experiments lead us to doubt, should be taken in great moderation. Vinegar, lemon juice, or such mild vegetable acid, though not necessary, may be added to some vegetables without apparent injury. Sugar is a concentrated form of nutriment, difficult to digest in large quantities itself, and having, like salt and vinegar, the power of preserving other substances not only from fermentation out of the stomach, but from digestion in it. Thus, fruit preserves are very hard of digestion, and must be eaten with great caution. Pepper, spices, mustard, and all heating and stimulating sauces, should be used very sparingly, if at all. Greasy food, melted butter, and pastry, are of difficult digestion.

Hot drinks debilitate the stomach, as the hot bath does the skin. Tea and coffee, like tobacco and ardent spirits, are narcotic poisons, which, for a time, stimulate, but finally weaken and destroy the nervous system. The best drink is *pure, soft, cold water.*

The nutriment in food should be mixed with a certain proportion of innutritious matter. In all fruits there is a proportion of woody fibre; also in roots, and in the bran of wheat and corn, and the skins and shells of other vegetables. The most perfect farinaceous food is unbolted wheat, either boiled or made into bread. Men can live very well on ten or twelve ounces of wheat a-day, with water for drink. Less wheat, with a portion of fruit, however, is better. Coarse wheat bread, or porridge, fruit, a little milk, make a beautiful and excellent diet. Maize is nearly as good as wheat—it may be even better for some constitutions. With it we can better do without milk or its products.

I add some tables, taken from standard authorities, which embody many important facts on diet. It is to be borne in mind that this system of living, besides being the most natural, the purest, the most beautiful, the healthiest, and the best, is also far the cheapest. No article of food costs so much, in soil, and labour, and care, as flesh. The corn given to a hog to fatten him, would feed a man more than ten times as long as the pork into which it is converted. There is no comparison for health and purity.

The following table presents the numbers expressing the composition of the principal kinds of food made use of, as well as that of flesh; thus affording a comparison of the nutriment of each article of vegetarian diet, with that of the flesh of animals.

The conclusions of this table are from the results of analyses by Playfair, and other chemists of established repute; and the separation of their parts of nutriment into flesh-forming principle, heat-forming principle, and ashes, is in relation to the necessary elements of food suited to the wants of the body, according to the views of the modern school of Chemistry, after Liebig.

WEIGHT.	ARTICLES OF DIET.	CONTAIN:		AND SUPPLY TO THE BODY:		
		Solid Matter.	Water.	Flesh-forming Principle.	Heat-forming Principle, with Innutritious Matter.	Ashes for the Body.
lb.		lb.	lb.	lb.	lb.	lb.
100	Turnips..........	11·0	89·0	1·0	9·0	1·0
"	Red Beet Root..	11·0	89·0	1·5	8·5	1·0
"	Carrots	13·0	87·0	2·0	10·0	1·0
"	Flesh..............	25·0	75·0	25·0	......	...
"	Potatoes..........	28·0	72·0	2·0	25·0	1·0
"	Bread (stale)	76·0	24·0	10.75	64·25	1·0
"	Peas............. ..	84.0	16·0	29·0	51·5	3·5
"	Wheat-meal.....	85·5	14·5	21·0	62·0	2·5
"	Beans......	86·0	14·0	31·0	51·5	3·5
"	Maize-meal	90·0	10·0	11·0	77·0	2·0
"	Oatmeal.........	91·0	9·0	12·0	77·0	2·0
"	Rice............. ..	92·4	7·6	8·4	82·0	2·0

The only direct evidence upon the digestibility of food in the human stomach, of indisputable import, is that published by Dr. Beaumont as the result of his observations in the case of Alexis St. Martin. The few following statements, expressing the digestibility of various articles of ordinary consumption in hours and minutes, are abstracted from the tables containing the results of his carefully conducted experiments:—

Articles of Vegetarian Diet.	H.	M.	*Articles of Flesh Diet.*	H.	M.
Soft Boiled Rice	1	00	Chicken Broth	3	00
Barley Soup	1	30	Roast Beef, Beefsteak	3	00
Boiled Tapioca, Barley, Milk	2	00	Chicken	3	15
Potatoes, Beans, Parsnips	2	30	Roast Mutton	3	15
Eggs (variously cooked)	2	37	Mutton Soup	3	30
Custard	2	45	Broiled Veal	4	00
Bean Soup	3	00	Roasted Duck	4	15
Bread (fresh)	3	15	Roasted Pork	5	15

In relation to the economy of vegetable food, Dr. Lyon Playfair stated, some years ago, at Drayton Manor, the residence of Sir Robert Peel, at a meeting of a great many distinguished men, that, "at London prices, a man may lay a pound of flesh on his body with milk for 3s., with turnips at 2s. 9d., with potatoes, carrots, butchers' meat without fat or bone, at 2s., with oatmeal at 1s. 10d., with bread, flour, and barley-meal, at 1s. 2d., and with beans at less than 6d."

It is calculated that fifteen persons may live on vegetable food, on the same land that would supply one with flesh. Some English estimates are more remarkable. Twelve acres are required to feed a man with beef alone; but on potatoes alone, he can live on the produce of one-ninth of an acre. Potatoes alone do not constitute a good diet, but millions have lived very well on potatoes and buttermilk. These facts throw a flood of light on the population question.

With a purely vegetarian diet, the Island of Great Britain, under thorough culture, could sustain one hundred millions of inhabitants. Now, a large part of the soil is wasted on cattle and game.

Another English estimate is given in the following table, which has many points of interest:—

ESTIMATED PRODUCE OF AN ACRE OF LAND.

	Per Year.	Per Day.
Mutton,............................	228 lbs.	10 oz.
Beef,.................................	182 ,,	8 ,,
Wheat,...............................	1,680 ,,	4½ lbs.
Barley,..............................	1,800 ,,	5 ,,
Oats,.................................	2,200 ,,	6 ,,
Peas,.................................	1,650 ,,	4½ ,,
Beans, ...	1,800 ,,	5 ,,
Rice,.................................	4,565 ,,	12½ ,,
Indian Corn,........................	3,120 ,,	8½ ,,
Potatoes, ...	20,160 ,,	55 ,,
Parsnips, ...	26,880 ,,	74 ,,
Carrots,.............................	33,600 ,,	92 ,,
Yams,................................	40,000 ,,	110 ,,
Turnip,..............................	56,000 ,,	154 ,,
Beet,.................................	75,000 ,,	205 ,,

"Adam Smith, in his *Wealth of Nations*, informs us: 'That the most beautiful women in the British dominions, are said to be, the greater part of them, from the lower ranks of the people of Ireland, who are generally fed with potatoes. The peasantry of Lancashire and Cheshire, also, who live principally on potatoes and buttermilk, are celebrated as the handsomest race in England.'

"The peasantry of Wales, Norway, Sweden, Russia, Denmark, Poland, Germany, Turkey, Greece, Switzerland, Spain, Portugal, and almost every country in Europe, from the most northern part of Russia to the Straits of Gibraltar, subsist principally, and most of them entirely, on vegetable food. The Persians, Hindoos, Burmese, Chinese, Japanese, the inhabitants of East Indian Archipelago, of the mountains of Himalaya, and, in fact, most of the Asiatics, live upon vegetable productions. The great body of the ancient Egyptians and Persians confined themselves to a vegetable diet; and the Egyptians of the present day, as well as the Negroes (whose great bodily powers are well known), live chiefly on vegetable substances. The brave Spartans, who for muscular power, physical energy, and ability to endure hardships, perhaps stand unequalled in the history of nations, were Vegetarians. The departure from their simple diet was soon followed by their decline. The armies of Greece and Rome, in the times of their unparalleled conquests, subsisted on vegetable productions. In the training for the public games in Greece, where muscular strength was to be exhibited in all its varied forms, vegetable food was adhered to, but when flesh-meat was adopted afterward, those hitherto athletic men became sluggish and stupid. ' From two-thirds to three-fourths of the whole human family, from the creation of the species to the present time, have subsisted entirely, or nearly so, on vegetable food, and always, when their alimentary supplies of this kind have been abundant, and of good quality, and their habits have been, in other respects, correct, they have been well nourished and well sustained in all the physiological interests of their nature.'

"LINNÆUS, one of the most celebrated naturalists that ever lived, speaking of fruits, says: 'This species of food is that which is most suitable to man; which is evinced by the series of quadrupeds, analogy, wild men, the structure of the mouth, of the stomach, and the hands.' M. DAUBENTON, the associate of Buffon, observes: 'It is, then, highly probable that man, in a state of pure nature, living in a confined society, and in a genial climate, where the earth required but little culture to produce its fruits, did subsist upon these, without seeking to prey upon animals.' GASSENDI, in his celebrated letter to Van Helmont, says: 'Wherefore I repeat, that from the primeval and spotless institution of our nature, the teeth were destined to the mastication, not of flesh, but of fruits.' Sir EVERARD HOME says: 'While mankind remained in a state of innocence, there is ground to believe that their only food was the produce of the vegetable kingdom.' BARON CUVIER, whose knowledge of comparative anatomy was profound, and whose opinion, therefore, is entitled to the greatest respect, thus writes: 'Fruits, roots, and the succulent parts of vegetables, appear to be the natural food of man; his hands afford him a facility in gathering them; and *his short, canine teeth, not passing beyond the common line of the others,* and the tubercular teeth, would not permit him either to feed on herbage, or devour flesh, unless these aliments were previously prepared by the culinary processes.' RAY, the celebrated botanist, asserts: 'Certainly, man by nature was never made to be a carnivorous animal, nor is he armed at all for prey or rapine, with jagged and pointed teeth, and crooked claws, sharpened to rend and tear; but with gentle hands to gather fruits and vegetables, and with teeth to chew and eat them.' Professor LAWRENCE observes: 'The teeth of man have not the slightest resemblance to those of carnivorous animals, except that their enamel is confined to their external surface. He possesses, indeed, teeth called canine; but they do not exceed the level of the others, and are obviously unsuited to the purposes which the corresponding teeth execute in carnivorous animals. * * * Thus we find, that whether we consider the teeth and jaws, or the immediate instruments of digestion, the human structure closely resembles that of the simiæ, all of which, in their natural state, are completely frugivorous.' Lord MONBODDO says: "Though I think that man has, from nature, the capacity of living either by prey or upon the fruits of the earth, it appears to me, that by nature, and in his original state, he is a frugivorous animal, and that he only becomes an animal of prey by acquired habit.' Mr. THOMAS BELL observes: 'The opinion which I venture to give has not been hastily formed, nor without what appears to me sufficient grounds. It is, I think, not going too far to say, that every fact connected with the human organisation goes to prove that man was originally formed a frugivorous animal, and therefore tropical, or nearly so, with regard to his geographical position. This opinion is principally derived from the formation of his teeth and digestive organs, as well as from the character of his skin, and the general structure of his limbs.'"

The natural drink—really the only drink of man—is water. Every mixture with it is of food or drugs. Wine, beer, etc., are alcohol, sugar, fruit, juices, etc., and water; but the water is the drink. The purer the water, the freer from animal, vegetable, and mineral admixture, the better. It is an entire mistake to think hard water better than soft. The water of Malvern is the purest and softest in England, and the most delicious. But there is no part of this country in which an abundant supply of pure soft water may not be had for drinking and culinary uses, by having proper cisterns. They should be large, tight, and built, if possible, of flat stones; but they may be made of brick, covered with cement. The water should pass into them through a filter, made of alternate layers of fine sand and charcoal, which may be renewed once a-year. No lead should be used about a cistern, as rain-water dissolves it, while spring or river water generally does not. The pipes should be wood, tin, or gutta percha. There is one cistern in Constantinople capable of supplying that vast city with water for sixty days. Perfectly soft and pure water may be obtained everywhere from hard or soft water, by distillation. All that is needed is a small still of iron or tinned copper, or even of common tin, with a tinned worm. Set over the kitchen fire, it will supply all the water for a family. The first water that passes over should be thrown away, and also the dregs. The water of the Malvern hills is simply rain water filtered through a pure vegetable loam, sand, and gravel.

Another condition of health is pure air. We can go for days without food, but not an hour without air. Respiration is the first act of independent life. We eat and digest at intervals, but we breathe continually. The stomach rests, but never the lungs. We need food every day, though not absolutely; but we must have air every minute. Air, then, of some kind, is a very vital necessity; and pure air, and plenty of it, is necessary to health.

The atmosphere is the great reservoir from which is obtained the most important materials of the organic world. It is a mixture of about four-fifths of nitrogen, one-fifth oxygen, from three to five ten-thousandths of carbonic acid, a trace of the nitrate of ammonia, and traces of phosphuretted and sulphuretted hydrogen. It also holds in solution a large quantity of water in vapour, which we see condensed into clouds, fog, dew, rain, etc. The atmosphere also contains and bears about odours of vegetables, and other aromal qualities, healthy and noxious. Of the latter are the miasms of intermittent and other forms of fever, and certain contagious diseases.

The relations of the atmosphere to man are various and important. Through the vegetable world it gives him food; it is the vehicle of sound; its weight or pressure is adapted to his organism; and he uses it in many mechanical appliances. But its great vital relation is to the blood, upon which it acts in the lungs, and through the skin.   The whole mass of the blood is constantly passing through the lungs, and so air is constantly brought into contact with the blood, in which it effects changes so important that life cannot go on without them.   The blood must have oxygen, and be freed from its carbonic acid, or it soon clogs and poisons the system.

At every inspiration we take in many cubic inches of air.   I have inhaled three hundred and twenty-five cubic inches at a single inspiration.   Ordinarily, it is said, we inhale about seventeen cubic inches.   When this air is expired, it contains less oxygen, more carbonic acid, and also various impure matters from the body.   Some persons' breaths are terribly diseased, and this is often the case with flesh-eaters, and those who do not bathe, while the breaths of vegetarians and water-cure people are often as sweet as the breath of cows, and so are those of all perfectly healthy persons.

If a man is shut in a close room, every breath he breathes changes the quality of the atmosphere. Minute by minute it grows impure.   It loses oxygen, becomes loaded with carbonic acid, and filled with excretory emanations both from the lungs and the skin.   Put many persons in the room, and this process is increased in rapidity.   In a railway carriage, steamboat, church, theatre, or concert-room, unless the greatest care is taken to ventilate them, by carrying off the foul air and admitting the pure, the atmosphere becomes totally unfit for respiration.   It is debilitating from its want of oxygen, deadly from its carbonic acid, and poisonous from the filthy emanations of people filled with all sorts of diseases.

A pure air, then, is of absolute necessity to the blood.   We must have quantity as well as quality.   If respiration is impeded in any way, it is a cause of disease.   The chest should be dilated to its utmost compass.   It must never be cramped by a stooping attitude. Every muscle of respiration must act with freedom. Neither the ribs, nor the muscles of the chest, nor the diaphragm, nor the muscles of the abdomen, which are the chief agents in expiration, should be in the least impeded by any dress or ligature.

By day and by night, at all times and in all places, sleeping and waking, we should have pure air, and breathe it plentifully. Of miasms, and other dele-terious qualities to be avoided, I shall speak furthe1 on when treating of the causes of disease.

The principles and modes of ventilation are very simple. Whenever the air in a room is warmer than the outer air, a crevice, ever so narrow, at the top of a window, will ensure a rapid change. Two currents are instantly formed—an upper one of warm air leaving the room, and a lower one of fresh air taking its place.

Fresh air must also come into every room to take the place of the air which goes up the chimney. But in every house, in cold weather, the air for every room should be warmed before it comes into the rooms, which could easily be done by proper furnaces.

Next to food and air, as conditions of health, comes exercise. I use this word here in a wide sense. By it I mean the activity of all voluntary functions. These are placed under the law of exercise, and depend upon it for the integrity of their life.

As development of every organ is necessary to the harmony of the system—that is, to health—and as exercise is necessary to development, it follows that exercise is one of the most important conditions of health.

Nature provides us air and food. These a man may have in isolation. Robinson Crusoe, on his desert island, could breathe the purest air, and live upon the most delicious fruits; he could take all needful bodily exercises, and could find use for some of his mental powers in the study of nature. But he had no exercise for the higher passions of the soul. These demand society. On the exercise of these, all the most exquisite enjoyments of his life depend. A man must have the exercise of benevolence, of friendship, of ambition, of familism, of love. To have these, he must have society, extensive and varied enough to gratify all these passions in all their various developments. The soul pines, and withers, and dies in isolation. And as the soul suffers, the body also becomes weak and diseased. Our muscles become wearied with inaction; we long to use them, but by long disuse, they at last lose their power. So of the passions. We long to love and to be loved; we long for the sweet accords of friendship, and the inspiring stimulus of ambition; these longings are the weariness and *ennui* of the soul. Those who do not know their own natures, feel vague yearnings; those who have studied them more carefully, have more definite desires. These longings of the soul must be satisfied, or we can have no spiritual health, and the body reflects the soul.

In the world, as it is, all exercise, and, consequently, all development, is fragmentary. The blacksmith and the boatman have large arms, the dancer has fine legs, the musician is all tune, the painter all form and colour, an artist is nothing but an artist, a politician is but a politician, the man of fashion is a mere dandy. There is no complete human being anywhere. There is sharpness, and even force, in particular directions, but no integral development and universality of power. Where is the man who is all he should be in himself and in his relations to God, and nature, and society? Where is the woman, strong, beautiful, self-centred, brave, religious, honest, kind, friendly, loving, wise, accomplished, with a true pride, and a noble ambition;

strengthening the weak, guiding the erring, animating the despairing, the life and soul of her sphere; great, and generous, and free?

In this word exercise lies the whole idea of education. A perfect analogy or harmony of action belongs to the whole system of animal organs, soul and body. Exercise gives both strength and facility of action. When we first sit down to the pianoforte how weak and bungling are our efforts to play. Day after day we accustom our fingers to obey the will, and to express the musical thought. Day by day it becomes easier to do so, and we soon learn to play rapidly, with ease, force, and expression, and without the least effort. The habit is formed. It is the same with every faculty and every passion. Every portion of the brain is susceptible of education, of gaining strength and facility by exercise, of forming good habits. Goodness is as habitual to the good as wickedness is to the wicked. It is as easy for men to be habitually brave, generous, noble, and just, as to be craven, stingy, mean, and dishonest. Men's hereditary character comes from the education of their ancestry; and in time it may be changed by the same agencies.

What men and women need for health are varied employments and amusements, attractive industry, pleasant society, the exercise and satisfaction of varied tastes, talents, and ambitions. All that can give happiness to man, promotes his health; all that can give health, promotes his happiness. Everywhere there is this reciprocal action, based upon the simplest laws. "Evils to man, and evils to man only, are sins against God." God can ask nothing of man but what is for his happiness; whatever promotes the happiness of man is therefore, pleasing to God. "Therefore, whether ye eat, or drink, or whatever ye do, do all to the glory of God."

Health demands, as its necessary conditions, then,

such parentage, birth, and blood, as shall secure a good, sound, well-developed constitution—"a sound mind in a sound body." It demands a pure and natural nutrition, or the observance of the laws of diet. It demands a pure air, or an observance of the laws of respiration. It demands the regular performance of all the organic and animal functions, secretions, excretions, and all muscular, nervous, intellectual, moral, and passional activities, which I have included in the law of exercise. It demands for the whole skin the cleanliness of daily ablution, without which its functions are not well performed. It demands a temperature neither so warm as to debilitate, nor so cold as to chill and stupefy; and for this purpose the clothing must be such as comfort requires, without impeding motion, aeration, or perspiration.

Dress, with many persons, and with all who are truly developed, is an art and a passion. Aside from comfort in regard to temperature; aside from its protection of our personality from those we have no sympathy with, and whose sight of our naked forms would be a profanation, dress is a mode of the expression of our sense of the becoming, the harmonious, and the beautiful, in texture, form, and colour. It is a language, a mode of life, a genuine out-growth of our natures, and is, therefore, a true necessity and a great enjoyment. Dress is, with many persons, a condition of health or a cause of disease. I do not speak of the vulgarities of tight lacing, nor the fettering absurdities of long skirts, sweeping the streets and crushing the spine; but of dress as beautiful or ugly, becoming or incongruous, harmonious or discordant. Be sure that an ugly, ill-fitting dress is a real cause of disease, and that a beautiful dress is both a cause and an indication of health.

The first quality of clothing is its cleanliness, the second is its comfort, the third is its fitness to our ɔrm, age, employment, and condition; the fourth is its beauty and spiritual harmony. The dress becomes a part of our being.

Rest, and especially the rest of sleep, is a condition of health. The animal organs demand rest and restoration. Recreation from a change of employments and enjoyments is not enough. There must be absolute repose. The whole brain must rest, probably from a necessity connected with its nutrition. Nothing exhausts and prostrates us sooner than the want of sleep. Sound sleep is the sign as well as condition of health. The infant, when its mental powers are just beginning to act and get quickly wearied, sleeps nearly all the time. In childhood and youth we sleep ten or twelve hours of the twenty-four. In maturity we find eight hours sufficient, and in old age we do with less.

Sleep is full or partial, and in partial sleep we have strange combinations of memory and fancy, and sometimes of our higher powers of thought and intuition. In these dreams also, and visions of the night, when the senses are locked up in a semblance of death, our souls seem to be opened to the influences of higher states of being.

Sleep is made unhealthy by indigestion, bodily weariness, mental excitement, or inquietude, by disordered passions and unsatisfied desires; by bad air, too much or too little clothing, by that which shuts in perspiration, by a bed too hard or soft, and by all unnatural conditions. As we spend, at least, one-third of our lives in sleep, we may as well take a little care how we sleep, and who we sleep with; for it is a condition of health, that we sleep with a healthy and congenial person, if with any. We must sleep with those we love, and not with those we hate, or who are in any degree repulsive to us. We must not sleep with those who are diseased, unless we are willing to give them our strength. The young must not sleep with the aged; it is too great a draft on their vitality. Children may sleep with the strong and mature, for there is a reciprocation of benefits. We radiate our lives, and partake of the radiations of others; but if we give much, and get little, we must be the losers. Men have a natural and proper repugnance to sleeping with each other, and so have many women, but not so much. In natural philosophy, like electricities repel, unlike attract. Physiology, or the science of nature, teaches us the conditions of health for every organised being. "Follow nature," was the true maxim of the old philosophers. We despise it for its simple brevity; but it contains all, and all that I have written, or could write in a thousand ages, on health or disease, would be but an amplification and illustration of this apothegm.

CHAPTER XIV.

THE CAUSES OF DISEASE.

DISEASE, in the sense in which I shall use it, as including also disorder, is the opposite, or the lack of health. It is "Any deviation from health, in function or structure, the cause of pain or uneasiness, distemper, malady, sickness, disorder, any state of a living body in which the natural functions of the organs are interrupted or disturbed, either by defective or preternatural action, without a disrupture of parts by violence, which is called a *wound*. The first effect of a disease is uneasiness or pain, and the ultimate effect is death. A disease may affect the whole body, or a particular limb or part of the body. We say a diseased limb, a

disease of the head or stomach, and such partial affection of the body is called a local or topical disease."

But the system is so bound up in common relations
of sympathy, that no disease can be entirely local. The
prick of the finest needle affects the whole system; and
a very slight wound may bring on death by lockjaw. If
there is any want of harmony in body or mind, it is disease. If there is inaction of any function, irregularity,
excess, or any kind of discordance, it is a disease.

And as the great sign and result of health is pleasure
or happiness, so the great symptom and effect of disease is pain or misery. And as we have pleasure in
all degrees, from the simplest feeling of satisfaction to
the keenest ecstasy, so we have all degrees of pain,
from uneasiness to agony.

Diseases are divided by pathologists into general
and local; but as there is no local disease which does
not affect the whole system, so it is believed by many
that there is no so-called general disease which has not
some special locality, throwing the force of its morbid
action upon some particular organ, either on account
of its weakness, its excited condition, or some peculiar
aptitude to receive it. Thus we have fevers, which
are considered general diseases of the nervous system or the circulation, becoming brain fevers, lung
fevers, bilious fevers, etc., according to the organ most
affected.

Diseases are also divided into functional and organic.
They are called organic, when some injury to, or alteration of the organ is perceptible; and functional, when
it is not. Where there is organic disease, there must
always be functional; where there is functional, there
must be organic disease somewhere, though not necessarily in the part which appears to be affected. It may
be in the nervous centres connected with it. Thus
asthma may be an affection of the spinal cord; and
irregular action of the heart, in most cases, comes from

some nervous connection with the stomach or generative organs.

Diseases are called sporadic, endemic, and epidemic; sporadic, when they appear in single cases at irregular intervals; endemic, when of constant occurrence from local causes; epidemic, when numbers of cases arise in the same district from some causes of temporary occurrence.

Diseases are acute, when recent and violent; chronic, when of long continuance, and slower progress; mild, when most cases recover; and malignant, when a large proportion are fatal; contagious, when they spread in any manner by the influence of the sick upon the well; otherwise, non-contagious. Highly contagious diseases are called virulent.

Disease, in any part, may be characterised by increase, or diminution, or irregularity of function, or some morbid change in its results. Thus, in the bowels there may be diarrhœa, or constipation, or each in alternation, or unnatural excretions; and the same of other organs. The heart may act with excessive force and rapidity; or it may be weak and rapid, or weak and slow, or irregular.

In inflammation there is preternatural heat, swelling, redness, pain. These symptoms, if diffused over the system, mark the state we call fever. Inflammation is a local fever; fever, a general inflammation.

Medical books are filled with the names of vast numbers of diseases, as a precisely similar affection of each organ of the body receives a corresponding name. Thus we have encephalitis, meningitis, arachnitis, parotitis, otitis, iritis, glossitis, pharyngitis, laryngitis, tracheitis, bronchitis, pleuritis, pericarditis, carditis, gastritis, enteritis, peritonitis, hepatitis, nephritis, cystitis, etc., etc., and all these hard words ending in ITIS, mean simply an inflammation of the brain, its membranes, the parotid gland, ear, tongue, throat, etc. The laws of one of these affections govern all. Everywhere we have nearly the same phenomena, the same causes, and similar modes of treatment.

All disease is attended by a lack of nervous energy, or the presence of morbid matter in the system, or both combined. In either case it may be hereditary or acquired, general or local, acute or chronic, mild or malignant. The causes of disease will best explain its nature; and by these we are directed to the means of cure.

The cause of a disease is, in many cases, scarcely to be separated in idea from the disease itself. Perhaps the word disease is applied more strictly to the phenomena which this cause produces, or to the efforts of the system to work against, overcome, or cast out the cause. If the system sank quietly and unresistingly under every cause of disease, we should scarcely know what sickness is. The pain and action of disease are the outcries and efforts of nature for relief.

A primary cause of disease is a hereditary lack of vitality. In such cases there may be early abortion, miscarriage, still-birth, death in infancy, marasmus, or lack of nutrition, rickets, convulsions, hydrocephalus, difficult dentition, and all the effects of general debility. There is the hereditary taint of scrofula, producing imperfect development, diseases of the skin, tubercular disease of the glandular system, tubercle of the brain, consumption of the lungs or bowels, tabes mesenterica, white swelling, hip disease, and the whole train of scrofulous disorders.

Other diseases are also hereditary, caused by the transmission of morbid matters, as gout, psora, salt rheum, syphilis, insanity.

A bad atmosphere, the crowd-poison of large towns and cities, produces cholera infantum, typhus, and lung diseases. Wherever people are crowded together, without cleanliness, the air becomes pestiferous. Infants die, all are debilitated; and when some other cause of disease is added, some miasm or contagion, these people are the victims. They die of typhus, or cholera, or dysentery; and are continually dying prematurely of consumption.

Diseased food—as the flesh of diseased animals; the milk of distillery fed cows; fish and flesh in the process of putrefaction; sausages, made of offensive materials; measley pork; narcotic and stimulating drinks; beer and porter, made worse by drugs; tobacco—these are all prolific causes of disease.

Uncleanly habits, wearing filthy clothes, the neglect of daily bathing, also tend to clog the pores, prevent the throwing out of effete, waste, and morbid matters, and cause the re-absoption of matters already expelled, and are fruitful causes of disease.

As all the functions of life are carried on by the nervous energy, a loss of that is not only a direct cause of functional debility, but by diminished vigour of excretion, it prevents the waste matter being carried out of the system; and this matter, thus retained, acts as a poison, and is a cause of almost every kind of disease. This reacts again; exhaustion causes impurity, and impurity produces exhaustion.

Consequently, anything which exhausts the power of the organic and animal system—anything which destroys the nervous energy, is in many ways a cause of disease.

Intense labour, care, and anxiety, protracted watchings, domestic unhappiness, any source of grief, may exhaust the nervous energy, and be a cause of disease. Sedentary employments, or monotonous labours, overtasking one set of organs and leaving the others without employment, may have the same effect.

The undue, and, therefore, disordered activity of any passion or appetite, is a cause of disease, by turning aside or exhausting the nervous energy that should be given to the whole system. Inordinate eating and drinking, avarice, ambition, all single and excessive passions, destroy the equilibrium of the system. But there is no passion so exhausting as amativeness. Its abuses are in proportion to its uses. The nervous exhaustion from its excess is the cause of most cases of dyspepsia, rheumatism, consumption, palsy, epilepsy, apoplexy, the nervous and uterine diseases of women, and, in fact a large proportion of all the diseases of mankind.

The abuse of amativeness, which sometimes begins in childhood, and even in infancy, rapidly exhausts the nervous power. The generative function takes strength from the organic and the animal powers. The stomach cannot digest, for want of the nervous energy so wasted. Nutrition cannot be carried on in the capillary system; the waste matter, which should be carried off by the secreting and excreting organs, is retained to poison the fountains of life; the skin becomes dry and withered; the eye dull; the mind weak and disordered; all noble feelings lose their force; the whole system falls into weakness and disorder; and then comes spinal disease, palsy, or some form of consumption.

Self-pollution in boys leads to involuntary seminal emissions, which, if frequent, are a serious disease, and continual cause of nervous exhaustion and impotence. In girls the same habit causes leucorrhœa, whites, irregular, profuse, and painful menstruation, falling of the womb, a loss of all pleasure in the sexual relation, difficult and painful childbirth, and a whole train of nervous and hysterical affections, which make the lives of women a burden to themselves and to all around them.

Amative excesses, even in mature age, and under lawful conditions, produce exhaustion, and so cause disease. Good, pious, loving husbands and wives kill each other with kindness, make their lives wretched, and give birth to short-lived, suffering children. In monotonous absorption in each other, they destroy each other; each, perhaps, falsely imagining that the other demands such murderous excess. Alas! how many stones can be seen in every church-yard, marking the graves of such husbands, and especially such wives, who add to these continuous excesses of ama tiveness, the exhaustion of gestation and childbirth. Such women marry at fifteen or twenty, and die before they are thirty-five.

The exhaustion of unnatural, or disordered, or excessive amativeness leads to cravings for stimulants. Men resort to tea, coffee, brandy, tobacco; they crave the richest and most stimulating food. These, in turn, provoke the action of the generative organs, and so the mischief goes on, until poor nature sinks in utter exhaustion; some disease sets in, and death relieves the sufferer from a body he has so much abused.

The stimulants I have just mentioned, whether taken to relieve this or any other debility, are all exhausting to the nervous system, from the reaction of their stimulating effects, and they are also poisons, which are retained in the system, acting upon the nerves, and a direct cause of disease. The concentrated extracts of tea, coffee, and tobacco, will kill small animals like so much prussic acid. Tobacco is one of the most insidious and debilitating of narcotics, stupefying and gradually weakening the nervous system. When used by the young its tendency is to stupefy the brain and bring on early impotence.

The craving for flesh, on account of its stimulating qualities, is another result of nervous exhaustion. A flesh diet is exciting, feverish, inflammatory, as well as impure, and often poisonous. Flesh, after long disuse, intoxicates like brandy. It has been found, by experiment, that chyle made of flesh putrefies in much less time than that made from vegetable sub-.

stances, and the same is notably the case with the blood. Flesh-eaters are especially subject to inflammatory diseases, particularly fevers and dysentery. A vegetable diet, based on physiological principles, with other healthy conditions, may be considered an absolutely certain safeguard against fevers, bowel complaints, cholera, small pox, and similar diseases.

The poisonous nature of animal matters in process of decomposition is shown by the following experiment of Magendie: "If we introduce into the jugular vein of a dog a few drops of water which has remained a little time in contact with animal substances in a state of putrefaction, in the course of an hour after the introduction, the animal will be depressed and lie down. Soon he will be attacked with an ardent fever; will vomit black and fœtid matter; his alvine evacuations will be similar; the blood will have lost its power of coagulation, will be extravasated into the tissues, and death will soon follow."

Flesh-eating, giving us an unnatural, excited life, leads to sensuality; sensuality brings exhaustion; exhaustion demands stimulation; and so the work of destruction goes on.

Dress may be a cause of disease, and an aggravation of other causes. Too much clothing weakens the skin, and keeps back the insensible perspiration. The compression of the female waist, by which the action of the diaphragm is destroyed, all the muscles of the respiration weakened, and the lungs, heart, liver, stomach, spleen, and pancreas compressed into one-half the space designed for them, is too evident a source of disease to require a word of comment.

Ligatures on any part of the body interfere with the freedom of the circulation; and tight boots and shoes are a great evil, from this cause, and from the compression of the nerves.

Any article of dress that excludes air and light from

the skin, that prevents the free circulation of the blood, that keeps in, or retains for re-absorption, the matter of perspiration, is a cause of disease. Great mischiefs, therefore, are occasioned by the use of water-proof hats, caps, and boots, and of oil-cloth or india-rubber, worn upon the person.

Changes of dress, from thick to thin, and in females, from the high-necked morning-dress to the bare arms, neck, and bosom of the evening, are causes of disease. Either, worn habitually, might answer. The lighter dress may be really the best; but when the skin has been weakened, and made sensitive, it will not bear these sudden changes.

Chill, from any cause, unless it is succeeded by immediate re-action and warmth, is a cause of disease. The sudden constriction of the skin by cold suspends its action; the matter it was expelling is thrown upon the mucous membrane in the throat, lungs, or bowels, and we have the feverish excitement and increased and morbid secretions which we call a cold, catarrh, diarrhœa, etc. Fresh and pure air is a necessary of healthy life, but a current of cold air when we are too weak to resist it, causes a sudden closing of the pores, and often leads to serious disorder.

Indolence, or lack of exercise of body or mind, is both an effect and a cause of disease. Laziness is often a real disease; which, however, may be overcome and cured by a resolute and habitual activity.

Attitude may be a cause of disease. Stooping distorts the spine and compresses the lungs, heart, stomach, etc. It interferes, therefore, with innervation, respiration, circulation, digestion, and disturbs, directly or indirectly, all vital processes. This habit is acquired in many monotonous employments; but a little care and resolution will prevent it, or even cure it where the habit is fully formed. Any crooked person may straighten himself, if he resolutely sets about it. Let him stand against the wall and straighten himself a dozen times a-day, continuing the effort at his work, in walking, and even in bed, and he will soon be as straight as a sapling. Any constrained and unnatural attitude may be a cause of disease.

Lack of light is a cause of disease in vegetables and animals. Light is the source of life; darkness is the synonym of death. All dark places are full of disease. Fashion, which turns day into night, by darkening sitting and drawing-rooms, and which substitutes the ghostly glare of gas and candles for the vital radiance of the sun, makes us look like blanched celery or potato vines growing in a cellar. Light is so absolute a condition of health, that its deprivation is always a cause of disease. Miners, men employed below decks on steamers, those who work in ill-lighted factories and cellars or at night, artists who exclude light from their studios, all suffer from the absence of this most direct expression of the Infinite Life.

Occupations are causes of disease, by their exhaustion, their monotony, their deprivation of healthy conditions, their slavery, and the utter hopelessness of improvement. With monotony, desperation, and bad conditions, whole ships' crews get the scurvy. In similar states, manufacturing populations sink under typhus and consumption. Many employments also introduce morbid matters into the system. Millers, stone-cutters, grinders, cotton-ginners and spinners, mattress-makers, bakers, etc., are subject to affections of the throat and lungs. Painters, gilders, and all workers in lead, arsenic, mercury, etc., are poisoned. It is certain death to work in a white-lead factory, or a mine of quicksilver. The manufacturers of some drug poisons, given as medicines, are soon destroyed by their inhalation and absorption.

The excessive and subversive actions of the passions are causes of disease. People die of disappointed love and ambition. Anger, grief, and even violent joy produce apoplexy, delirium, hysteria, hemorrhage. Fear acts on the circulation, turns the hair white in a few hours, brings on premature old age, and even kills suddenly. Sorrow, care, anxiety, jealousy, produce the same effects less rapidly. All discord of the passions is disease.

Disease of the mind is reflected upon the bodily organs; and so it is called a cause of disease, when it is only an extension. Love and its subversions act upon the heart and lungs; other passions upon the stomach, liver, kidneys, and bowels.

Poisons taken into the system by the stomach, the lungs, or through the skin, or which act directly upon the nervous system, are among the most frequent causes of disease.

All the waste matter of the body, arising from the action and consequent disintegration, combustion, or destruction of all the tissues, which are continually renewed by nutrition, becomes, if retained in the system, a cause of disease, a real virus, a true poison. This is known to be true of urea, or the solid matter of the urine, the bile, the fæcal matter, the matter of perspiration, and the carbon excreted by the lungs. Any interruption of the functions of skin, liver, kidneys, intestines, or lungs, is, therefore, a cause of disease by the retention of morbid matter.

Similar matter taken in food, and especially in eating the carcases of dead animals, which always contain it, is a cause of disease. The introduction of a certain quantity of this matter of putrefaction taints the breath, and overtasks all the purifying organs. These poisons may be drunk in impure water, and are also inhaled in crowded atmospheres, and absorbed by contact with uncleanly persons. Plagues, camp-fevers, jail-fevers, typhus, dysenteries cholera, and many

other diseases, are either solely caused or greatly aggravated by this animal poison.

Of a similar character is the effluvia from grave-
yards, which poison all around them.   Portions of
London were formerly pestiferous from this cause.

The poison of animal putrefaction is sometimes so
virulent, that the slightest inoculation with it, by the
prick of a needle, or the cut of a scalpel, produces
death.   Many surgeons and medical students have
died of such inoculations.

Tea, coffee, alcohol, opium, tobacco, all stimulants,
and all narcotic poisons in habitual use, are causes
of disease, both by the stimulation and consequent
exhaustion of the nervous system, and by their presence, as morbid or diseasing matters in the system.
The system of an old tea or coffee drinker becomes
saturated with these infusions.

Alcohol fills all the tissues of the inebriate, so as
sometimes to render his whole body a subject of
spontaneous combustion.   In the water-cure, we have
patients from whom opium and tobacco are thrown
out for weeks together, in such quantities as to stain
sheets and bandages and poison the atmosphere around
them.

Closely allied to these, as causes of disease, are the
poisonous drugs administered as medicines.   And it
must not be forgotten that syphilis, scrofula, and probably every kind of blood-poison, can be taken by
vaccination, which, so far from being a protection
against small-pox, seems to have been one of the
chief causes of the late epidemics.   It is never safe to
take matter from another body into our own.   We
risk taking all its diseases.   There is no doubt that
thousands have been mortally poisoned by vaccination, made compulsory by law upon the whole population.   Apparently healthy children have scattered
hereditary syphilis, and, perhaps, even worse diseases.

Stimulants weaken the parts they excite; tonics destroy tone; cathartics produce constipation; mercury, quinine, arsenic, antimony, and opium, are poisons, remaining in the system for years, and wrecking the strongest constitutions. The quack medicines which deluge the country are mischievous just in the ratio of their potency. The sassafras and molasses, which costs sixpence, and is sold for a dollar a bottle as sarsaparilla, cannot do much harm, unless it contains, as it commonly does, a minute but effective portion of arsenic or corrosive sublimate.

Causes of disease exist in the water we drink. Hard water, containing lime in some of its combinations, or other mineral matter, is totally unfit for drinking, and is the cause of gravel, stone, goitre, and other morbid growths, and is also a common cause of dyspepsia and bowel complaints. Hard water, that will not wash the skin, nor penetrate and soften food in cooking, is not fit for drink, and scarcely for bathing. Wherever the water of springs or wells is hard, rain water should be caught in large, clean cisterns, and carefully preserved for all domestic uses. Filtered through alternate layers of sand and charcoal, it is the purest and sweetest water we can have. It is even better to take the trouble of distilling water, than to use such as is hard.

Water containing vegetable and animal impurities, and animalculæ, may introduce morbid matters into the system. Fresh, cold spring water, or clean, well-preserved rain water, however, contains no animal life. Water, to contain animalculæ, must have been exposed to light and warmth, and contain, also, some vegetable or animal matter. Water infiltrated with sewage, and containing decaying animal matter, is a fertile cause of disease. One well, into which filth can percolate, may breed cholera or typhus in a whole district. All doubtful water should be thoroughly filtered, or boiled, or both.

Causes of disease, of more or less potency, are found in the atmosphere, in what is called *malaria*, which simply means bad air, but is used to designate the unknown cause of many endemic and epidemic diseases. There seems much reason to believe that some of these diseases are caused by telluric or aromal causes, so subtle as not to be influenced by atmospheric changes and motions.

Carbonic acid gas, if a poison, is still more a mechanical cause of illness or death. In a well, a mine, or a close room, it displaces the atmosphere, and produces asphyxia, by hindering us from breathing. We drown in this heavy gas, as in water. In each case we die for want of breath. It kills us just as it puts out a candle, by preventing the access of oxygen. A well is freed from it by putting in quick-lime, which absorbs it in being converted into a carbonate. The means of resuscitation are the same as in drowning, only that cold water may be dashed over the body, while after drowning we try to restore warmth.

In a crowded, close room, the oxygen is soon exhausted, and the air filled with carbonic acid, besides much diseased matter. A fashionable singer orders her concert-rooms to be shut close, and ladies are carried out fainting. All suffer from want of breath and poisoning. Every one's health is diminished and their lives shortened. Judges, lawyers, and jurymen, are murdered in the wretchedly ventilated court-rooms of England in the same manner. Clergymen and their congregations are all made sick. In 1756, one hundred and forty-six Englishmen were confined one night in an East Indian dungeon, called the Black Hole of Calcutta: one hundred and twenty-three—all but twenty-three—perished before morning. Nearly a century afterward, seventy-five human beings perished in one night, by being fastened, during a gale, in the close cabin of an English steamer

The malaria which seems to be the cause of typhus fever, dysentery, camp fever, jail fever, ship fever, yellow fever, appears to be the putrid and poisonous exhalations of either decaying vegetable or animal matter, or of uncleanly and diseased living persons. These diseases are therefore contagious—that is, each sick person helps to poison the atmosphere that produces or determines the disease. Decaying vegetables, or putrid bilge water in the hold of a ship, or in a cellar on shoré, will cause fever. The opening of a drain in certain localities, has caused attacks of cholera in a street which was considered quite healthy. The causes of yellow fever are circumscribed to particular localities. A grove of trees, or even a high fence, is a barrier. A ship with yellow fever, at quarantine, has given the disease to persons residing at the leeward.

But whatever the nature of these causes, there seems to be some specific agency which determines the nature of the disease. With the same kind of persons, suffering from the same causes, we have at one time dysentery; at another, erysipelas; at another, hospital gangrene; at another, typhus, or ship, or jail fever; at another, yellow fever; at another, cholera. We have also special animal poisons determining to measles, scarlatina, small-pox, etc.

We have also the malaria which causes intermittent fever, or fever and ague. This disease is attributed to decaying vegetation, but it is found in deserts, and is wanting in the most fertile localities. Stagnant water is said to cause it, but we find it on dry prairies, and miss it amid swamps and morasses. Localities which seem to the observer precisely similar, and even but a few miles apart, are entirely different in this respect. Any disturbance of the soil, as digging a canal, or grading a railroad, may bring out the poison. The cause seems to be in the soil, and not in decaying matter. either animal or vegetable. It is not found on

certain geological strata, nor above a certain degre
of latitude. As we go south it is more intense, and is
combined with other malaria to produce remittent
fevers. The malaria of the Carolina rice swamp, or
of the African coast, is almost certain death to a white
man from a single night's exposure. By day the rarefi-
cation of the air, or the direct action of the sun, either
disperses or neutralises the poison.

Liability to disease varies in individuals, according
to several circumstances. In every community, exposed to the same general causes of malaria, contagion,
etc., some are well, some sick, some die. For all this
there must be a reason. Those who have the most
vitality, the most power of resistance, the least predisposition to disease, who have been born and are living
in the most healthy conditions, are proof against outward causes of disease. They pass through plague,
yellow fever, cholera, and all ordinary epidemics
unharmed. The cholera is a good illustration of this.
There can be no doubt that its specific, determining
cause was over the whole city of New York, but its
victims were among those who were weakened by
other causes, and were living in unhealthy conditions. Of the 5,000 who died of cholera in New
York in 1849, 3,000 were buried in the Roman Catholic cemetery. They were mostly poor Irish and
Germans, living crowded together, in the most unhealthy parts of the city, and surrounded by many
causes of disease. The other two thousand were
exhausted by intemperance, by sensuality, or in some
way unable to resist the diseasing influence. There
was no danger to any really healthy person. And
this is true of most external causes of disease. In proportion to the energy of our vitality and the purity of
our lives, is our power to resist and overcome diseasing
influences.

The rate of mortality from bad water, other filth,

over-crowding, and similar causes of disease, on the
east side of London, is double that on the west, or
aristocratic side. From twenty to thirty thousand
poor labouring people in London are killed every
year by filth alone; while the number of those who
are sick of fever is twelve times as great.

In the healthiest parts of London the deaths by
cholera were 8 in 10,000. In the worst parts, 225 in
10,000. Had London been perfectly healthy, there
would have been 0 in 10,000.

There is another preventive to particular forms of
disease, in that power of the system to adapt itself to
unusual and even unnatural conditions, which may be
called the power of habit or acclimation. Persons get
accustomed to the malaria of yellow fever, for instance.
Habit enables a man to take twenty grains of opium
at a dose; when he began, five grains would have
killed him. Custom enables a man to smoke or chew
tobacco all day long; when he began, a single quid or
half a cigar made him deadly sick.

It is in this way that men bear so much evil, live in
filth, eat flesh, breathe foul air, use tobacco and whisky,
and become hardened to all the miseries of life. They
are acclimated. But the whisky, and malaria, and pork,
and medicine, and domestic broils, and tobacco, are
evils none the less, and they kill none the less, because
nature has the power of fortifying herself, and making
a protracted instead of a violent resistance.

For all acute diseases are the strong and rapid efforts
of nature to rid us of disease; while chronic diseases
are the weakened and slow efforts to the same end.
The causes of disease are of two kinds; weakness,
original; or by exhaustion of the nervous power or
vital energy; and the presence of diseasing matter in
the system. The latter may be hereditary, an effect,
or even a cause of the former. The presence of a sick
person will produce an effect of painful sympathy upon

an impressible person.   Even a letter coming a thous-
and miles, will produce on such a person, before it is
opened, such pain as the writer may have been suffering.   A magnetised ring or a lock of hair gives to some
persons a feeling of the mental states and bodily condition of an absent friend.   If I lay my hand upon the
region of Firmness, Self-esteem, etc., I give a feeling
of strength.   By an opposite influence, I produce depression and pain.   I have known persons to be thrown
into convulsions by the simple feeling of the spheres
of those about them.   The presence of a person of a
more congenial sphere, or in another state of feeling,
would restore them.

CHAPTER XV.

CURATIVE AGENCIES.

"PREVENTION is better than cure."   Even the ratio
in which it is better is sometimes set forth; and we
are told that "an ounce of prevention is worth a
pound of cure."   Doctors find that prevention is in
no demand, or that it is too cheap to afford them any
profit; for they do not deal in the article.   Quacks
advertise their nostrums as preventives of disease,
especially when there is some prevailing epidemic.
Doctors are generally in favour of vaccination, for
they are paid for it; and if disease, as many believe, is
thereby propagated, and even the small-pox but little,
if any, diminished, it is a profitable preventive.

How can diseases be prevented?   Simply in two
ways: by living, as far as possible, in accordance with
all the conditions of health; and by avoiding, in like
manner, every cause of disease.   By keeping up the

strength and purity of the system; by avoiding all excess, and every means of exhaustion; and by living so as to keep free from all matter of disease.

The cure of disease is not accomplished by any medical system. Nature does her own work. It is the power of life that moulds and builds up the organism; it is the intelligent soul that first forms the body, and presides over all its processes, which struggles against disease, overcomes it, and casts it out of the system. No device of man can accomplish such a work as this; and man's efforts to assist nature have, in most cases, been full of error and mischief.

In all cases of disease, when the vital force is sufficient, nature effects a cure. When there is more disease than this vital force can overcome, nature sinks under the effort, and the patient dies; sometimes after a violent and brief struggle, sometimes after a weak and protracted one. The well-meaning doctor, in many cases, instead of attacking the disease, if, indeed, he had any means to do so, begins a violent assault upon nature; he attacks and weakens the vital energy, using poison and steel against her, bleeding, blistering, and drugging, until he changes the whole aspect of affairs; and nature, who was strong enough to cope with disease, sinks under the united forces of disease and the doctor. Or it may be a drawn battle; nature, overpowered by drugs, gives up the struggle, and each party—nature, disease, and drugs—occupy the disputed territory, and patch up a peace. But this does not last long. Nature renews the struggle, the doctor renews his mischievous interference; and life is made a long agony by this intestine war.

When nature is left alone to cope with disease, the struggle is brief in proportion to its violence. The matter of disease is cast out by some sharp crisis—vomiting, diarrhœa, or sweating—and there is a quick recovery. I believe that a much larger proportion of

o

cases in all diseases would recover in this way than with the ordinary methods of interference.

If we understand the mode of cure adopted by nature, we can see how she may be aided by art. There is an intelligent soul which presides over the bodily organism, as a whole, and in every minutest part. When a bone is broken, or an artery tied, this intelligent power goes to work to repair damages. It is the same in all vital processes. When poison, as tobacco or opium, is taken into the system, there is at first a violent effort to cast it out by vomiting, preceded by nausea, or sickness at the stomach. In case of a failure to vomit, the next process is sweating. In one way or the other, or both, they are expelled, unless in too large a dose, when they overpower life, and cast it out of the body.

If poison or diseasing matter is taken into the system in so small quantities as not to call for any violent effort to expel it, it is treated just like a few persons who venture into an enemy's country. They are either allowed to go quietly out, by the usual avenues, or are made prisoners. Francke, a German pathologist and hydropathist, has made some curious observations on this point. He says, that in all cases where poison, or morbid matter, is not at once cast out of the system, it is enveloped in a coating of mucus, to prevent it from doing injury, and then either carried out by the usual processes, or, if this cannot well be done, it is retained in the system, each atom being thus "slimed up," and protected from doing more mischief.

But as these matters accumulate in the system, there is a constant tendency to drive them out; and every cold, every fever, every paroxysm of disease is such an effort. The matter is always there, and always liable to be dislodged, and to be the cause of diseased action, or of the effort toward health; but when nature fails, either from the weakness of her own power or the interference of the doctors, and the introduction of more poison, she either gives up the struggle finally, and retires from the body altogether, or spends her remaining efforts in again sliming up the *materies morbi*.

Sometimes masses of these slimed-up matters, medicines, and other poisons, are collected along the walls of the stomach and intestines, covering and rendering useless large patches of those organs. Sometimes they appear in the form of tubercle. In this case they have got as far as the glands, the lungs, the areolar tissue, and even to the skin. There are many phenomena in the cure of disease by hydropathy, which give, to say the least, a violent presumption of truth to this hypothesis.

But in whatever particular way nature deals with the matter of disease, whether the product of the system or introduced from without, the general fact is well ascertained, that these matters are sometimes cast out at once, and sometimes after a long course of years, during which they remain in the system, always oppressing it, and liable at any time to be a cause of disorder, like the aforesaid prisoners in an enemy's country.

We have, in the medical world, five schools of pathology—the nervous, solidist, the humoral, the chemical, and the mechanical. They believe, respectively, that all diseases arise from irregular nervous action, from disease of tissues, from humors in the blood, from chemical changes, and from animalcular or mechanical irritation. My pathology includes all these theories, and all the facts on which they are founded.

Modes of practice are based on these exclusive theories of disease. The nervists deal in sedatives, anti-spasmodics, and poisons, which directly affect the nervous system; the solidists rely on mercurial and other alteratives; the humorists bleed and purge; the chemists give alkalies and acids; and the animalculists strive to poison the enemy, forgetting, as an old doctor said of worm medicines, that man is but a worm, and is liable to be killed by the same poisons.

As diseases consist of exhaustion and impurity; as exhaustion causes impurity, and impurity produces exhaustion, two things are requisite to a cure. These two should be written in letters of gold—INVIGORATION and PURIFICATION.

Let me make this emphatic by two definitions:

Pathology.—Exhaustion and impurity resulting in disease and death.

Therapeutics.—Invigoration and purification resulting in health and life.

In each case a third term is wanting, which belongs to the domain of psychology, or the science of the soul. In pathology it lies back of exhaustion, and in therapeutics its curative agency must precede invigoration. The pathological term I shall call *inversion*, to express discordance of the soul. It is a condition of ignorance, unbelief, and desperation. The opposite psychical agency is one of insight, hope, faith, and loving confidence in nature and in God. It is a state of concordance or harmonisation. We may express the whole subject in this triple formula:

Physiology—Harmony in the soul; energy in the vital or nervous power; purity in the organism. Unity of God, man, and nature.

Pathology—Inversion in the soul; exhaustion of vital or nervous energy; impurity of organism. General disintegration.

Therapeutics—Harmonisation of the soul; invigoration of the vital or nervous energy; purification. Integral restoration.

The physiological condition is that of health, harmony, and fulness of life.

The pathological is one of disease, discordance, and dissolution.

The therapeutical is one of hope, effort, and restoration.

So united are the three terms of each condition, that each one may produce the two others; or if we can produce two, the third is almost certain to follow. The best or worst results, however, are derived from the concurrence of all three.

For instance, harmony in the soul gives energy of vitality and bodily purity. Energy of vitality purifies the body and harmonises the soul. Bodily purity gives energy of life and harmony of feeling.

Or, inversion or discord of the soul produces exhaustion and impurity. Exhaustion brings discord and impurity. Impurity brings discord and exhaustion.

On the other hand, harmonisation, or faith and hope, gives energy and purity. Invigoration inspires hope, and causes purification; and a simple bodily purification will go far to produce vigour of life and harmony of the spirit.

Here, then, in a few words, and simply stated, is my theory of Health, Disease, and Cure. Let us proceed to its practical application.

What agencies can we make use of safely and profitably, to aid nature in her three-fold work of cure? In the answer to this question lies the basis of all therapeutical science.

The first thing we must learn—the first principle of medicine, and the one oftenest disregarded, is to do no mischief. It is not true that *we must do something.* Unless we know what to do, it is always safer and better *to do nothing* If we are not sure that we can aid nature, we must not run the risk of hindering her with our interference. All experience shows that, in a great majority of cases, she effects a cure without assistance, and even in spite of mischievous efforts.

But the moment any one is taken ill—that is, the

moment nature begins the operation of expelling some matter of disease—everybody wants to be doing something to the patient. Every old woman rushes in with her infallible nostrum, and nature, who has honestly set to work to cure a disease, finds herself hindered on every side. When the stomach is incapable of digestion, it must be deluged with gruels, rice water, and barley water, as if the moment one was taken sick, he was in imminent danger of starvation. Then comes the doctor, and if one of the common sort, the attack begins in earnest. A few years ago out came the lancet, and followed its rude gash a quart of blood. Poor nature, feeling the work she had to do, and needing all her strength, gasped at this murderous sacrifice; but the next attack was to cover fifty square inches of the skin with a torturing blister, and at the same time to pour down the throat doses of the most virulent poisons of the *materia medica*. This process went on, and when nature finally sunk under the disease, and the added exhaustion of a vile and torturing medication, everybody consoled himself with the idea that "everything was done that could be done;" it should be added, "to kill the patient."

Napoleon, a man of grand intuitions, once said to the Italian physician, Antonomarchi: "Believe me, we had better leave off all these remedies. Life is a fortress which neither you nor I know anything about. Why throw obstacles in the way of its defence? Its own means are superior to all the apparatus of your laboratories. Covisart candidly agreed with me that all your filthy mixtures are good for nothing. Medicine is a collection of uncertain prescriptions, the results of which, taken collectively, are more fatal than useful to mankind. Water, air, and cleanliness are the chief articles in my pharmacopœia."

If medicine were only as wise as surgery! When man has broken a bone, the surgeon is content to put it in its place, prescribe rest, and a moderate diet, and leave nature to mend it. But when it is the liver or lungs that are disordered, the doctor bleeds, and blisters, and doses, gives alterative, cathartic, opiate, and does more mischief in a week than nature can remedy in a year. I have no patience with the folly of patients, or the ignorance, to call it no worse, of physicians. But when I see how the latter are educated, and the former deceived, I cannot wonder at the result. I have seen hundreds of medical students; I have attended the lectures of two medical colleges. " I speak what I know, and testify what I have seen." What Napoleon said is true of the highest and most enlightened. What, then, must be the truth respecting the great mass of medical practitioners?

But there are things that we may do, wisely, safely, and with good results. To know these, is the true science of medicine. To do nothing, is better than to do mischief; but it is not so well as to do something that should be done. When a man has fallen into a ditch, we had better do nothing than to jump upon him, and bury him deeper; but it is much better to carefully pull him out, cleanse him of the mud, put him in the right path, and send him on his way rejoicing.

We can do all that is practicable to remove the causes of disease, which must be ascertained by a thorough examination. Patients cheat physicians and even themselves, as to the causes of disease. How seldom will a woman confess to tight lacing, or a man to gluttony. We must not expect confessions of secret licentiousness. But we must do all in our power, and admonish the patient as to the existence of hidden causes of evil.

There are potent causes of disease that are not easy to remove. When a feeble, nervous woman is crushed, soul and body, by a brutal husband—I beg pardon of all honest brutes, but there is no other word—it is not so easy to take her away from him, or to send him away from her, and such cases are generally hopeless. The husband may be the only real cause of disease; and without a separation, there can be no cure. So of many false and oppressive social conditions. Children are oppressed by unsympathising parents; parents have their lives cursed by perverse children; vast numbers suffer from relatives on whom they are dependent. Some of the benefits which patients receive at water-cure establishments and other sanitary resorts, come from their having left such causes of disease behind them; but when they go back, they are too apt to relapse.

The common causes of exhaustion may generally be removed, unless they belong to the condition of the patient, such as his necessary avocations, care, trouble, etc.; or unless the disease itself is of an exhausting character, as leucorrhœa in women, and involuntary seminal emissions in men. We may change the diet, or interdict food entirely; we may remove the patient from bad air, or secure him ventilation; we may attend to external cleanliness.

In short, we may safely and rightly, as far as possible, give to the diseased the conditions of health; and in this we have done much for his restoration. In this, as in all other things, there is one grand rule of practice: *that we adapt our measures to the condition of the patient.*

"Cease to do evil, learn to do well," applies to sins bodily as well as sins spiritual. But what is well for the well man is not always well for the invalid. It is well for the well man to eat, drink, take exercise, labour, and partake of all enjoyments. But the best thing for the sick man may be to entirely stop eating, and to rest, mind and body. The effort to digest food, to take exercise, and to "keep up," is a cause of exhaustion. Many patients are injured by long walks, as well as by too much treatment. They are ambitious to cope with others in exercise: they want to get their money's worth of treatment; exhausted by both, they eat to get strength, and overtask again the digestive powers; finally they sink under this triple mischief, and go away worse than they came.

The hunger-cure, or absolute rest to the stomach, is one of the simplest means of cure, in most acute and dyspeptic diseases. No food, not one atom of any kind, should ever be taken in some cases of acute disease, until they are cured. Starve and drink water is all that is needed for the digestive apparatus. This, with cold water to the skin, for cooling and purification, and cold water injections to the bowels for the same purpose, are the means of cure.

And in all chronic diseases, which are dependent upon or complicated with dyspepsia, the whole digestive system needs rest, absolute rest, more than anything else. In many cases a patient should resolutely starve, not live on slops, but eat *nothing*, and drink water for three weeks, taking daily ablutions and injections, and it will go further to secure a cure than months of the most active treatment, when this is neglected. I have seen this tried, and know its efficacy. When the patient begins to eat, it should be the smallest quantity of food, and of the simplest quality; say one ounce of coarse bread, and two ounces of fruit a-day for the first week; then two ounces of bread and four of fruit for another week; then three ounces of bread and six of fruit for a month. By this time the worst dyspeptic will have digestion for meals progressively larger, until he reaches the standard of health, and his whole system will have undergone the most remarkable changes.

One of the best cures of dyspepsia I ever heard of was that of Mr. Robinson, of Nantucket, who cured himself by eating an ounce of dry, coarse, unbolted wheat bread, at a meal, three times a-day, drinking nothing but water. Sometimes at supper he only ate

half an ounce. He chewed this thoroughly, and persevered in this course for some months. At first he
lost flesh, but afterwards gained both flesh and strength,
and was soon able to perform the labour of a common
working farmer. He was thoroughly cured. I believe
the cure would have been still more rapid had he taken
the course I have recommended.

The world has one great agent of purification, and
that is water. It is the universal solvent. Entering
largely into the composition of all organic beings, it is
by its agency that all vital processes are performed.
It is the great agent of digestion, nutrition, and excretion. It is at once the vitaliser and purifier of the
world. The matter which is carried out of the system
is first dissolved in the watery portion of the blood.
Then it passes from the lungs dissolved in vapour,
from the skin in perspiration, from the kidneys in
urine, from the intestinal canal in fæcal evacuations,
which are poured into it through a million sluice-ways,
by the agency of water, which is again re-absorbed.
When impurities gather upon the surface, we wash
them off with water. This single agent, then, in its
simplest internal uses, affords us the means of one of
the most important conditions of cure, that of purification; and drinking pure water is alone sufficient in a
vast number of cases. Thirst is the call of the intelligent organism for water. It is a common symptom
of disease, and especially of all diseases of impurity,
rather than exhaustion. Nature commonly knows
what she requires. Water is wanted to dissolve the
impure matters in the system, and carry them off.
The copious drinking of soft water is alone often
sufficient to cure a fever. It is followed by profuse
sweating, large evacuations of urine, a full action of
the bowels; the system gets a thorough clearing out,
and the patient, after recovering from the fatigue of
this effort, is well.

The internal applications of water, in the cure of disease, are drinking, and injections by the rectum, and by the vagina. They all, when taken cold, answer the two great purposes of cure. They cleanse and invigorate. Injections into the rectum, penetrating, as they may, the entire length of the colon, soften accumulations of fæcal matter, and wash them away. In all cases of constipation, or where there is not a full daily action, these injections should be taken to the extent of from one to three pints, retaining them for some minutes, and repeating them as often as needed. Every person liable to sickness should have a good syringe for this purpose. The pump syringe is the best; but any kind will answer which will inject water into the bowels. There is scarcely any case of disease in which injections once or twice a-day may not be used to advantage. In diarrhœa they are taken cold after every discharge, to wash away corroding excretions, and to give strength to the part. In dysentery they cleanse, reduce inflammation, stop hemorrhage, and give tone or vigour. Injections of cool or cold water into the vagina, and upon the uterus by that means, produce the same effects cleansing, checking hemorrhage, and giving energy to the parts.

Water, applied externally, also produces all these effects. It purifies, cools, and invigorates every part to which it is applied. Try it on the hand. Try it when it is dirty, dry, hot, and wearied. Dip and rub it a few moments in cold water. It becomes clean, moist, cool, and invigorated. Try it on the whole body, and you will find the same effect.

This is a matter so important as to require a little more explanation.

Water cleanses by its power of dissolving substances.

Water cools by its coming in contact with so many points of surface, and its power of conducting heat, and often by evaporation. It cools the whole surface, or any part to which it is applied. Dipping the hands into cold water will cool the whole body.

Water reduces inflammation by lowering the temperature, equalising the circulation, and by cooling, contracting the capillaries, and driving the blood out of them. This contraction or constriction of the capillaries is also connected with an infusion of nervous power and quickened circulation, which contributes to a return of healthy action.

Water invigorates in many ways; by the very process of purification obstructions are removed, and the nervous energy allowed to act freely; by the equalisation of the circulation, the whole system acts in harmony, and its force is augmented by being well distributed; by the direct action of cold in quickening the action of the capillaries; by the re-action of the heat-forming power of the nervous system, quickening the circulation, especially in the capillaries, and developing vital heat, which seems to be only an expression of vital energy.

This last is a very curious matter. It seems to be governed by the general law of exercise. If we give a weak person a cold bath, or a wet sheet pack, he may be long in re-acting against it, or in getting warm. We carefully proportion the length of the bath or the quantity of the sheet to this re-active power. But, like other powers, it gains strength by exercise. Every day the patient re-acts better; and we find that the whole strength or vital energy increases with this power of re-acting against cold, until we have a restoration to health. This is the process of invigoration. It is a kind of vital gymnastics, or education of the organic powers.

We push the purifying process, and join it with the invigorating, by exciting the action of the skin by long packs in the wet sheet, or in dry blankets, followed by

a cold bath. We prolong the invigorating process in
the partial application of the sitz-bath; and both purification and invigoration are combined in the wet
jackets, bandages, and compresses.

Thus, water is the great agent of vigour and purity;
of the first, by its being so admirable a means of controlling temperature; of the second, by its solvent
power. It seems also to possess magnetic or electric
properties of a peculiar kind, which act upon the
nervous system; a kind of vitality, especially when
freshly drawn and living. Our own vitality is probably nourished by a great element of vitality in
nature, of which water is one of the mediums; and
hence its enlivening and invigorating influence.

Water has been considered the material corres-
pondent of the Divine Truth, and its effect upon the
body corresponds to that of truth upon the soul, purifying and invigorating.

Light can never be neglected as a curative agent,
or a condition of health. The sick are often shut up
in darkness. On the contrary, they should have an
extra share of light, and, if possible, bask in the direct
rays of the sun.

Animal magnetism, or the power which one person
has of strengthening the vitality of another, and controlling its action, may often be used with singular
advantage.

Congeniality, friendship, love, faith or trust, hope,
and joy, in all their expressions, should never be lost
sight of as remedial agents, giving vigour to the soul,
and influencing every bodily function.

This is the *materia medica* of nature. I shall now
describe more particularly the processes to be used in
the treatment of disease, with their applications, and
the errors to be guarded against. I wish to make these
directions so plain, that no reader of this book may
ever be obliged to write to me for further explanations.

CHAPTER XVI.

PROCESSES OF WATER CURE.

THE water used in most of the processes of water-cure should be fresh, soft, clean, and newly drawn. It should be soft, especially for drinking, and soft water is better for bathing; but hard or salt water, if cold and living, has less cleansing, but abundant invigo-rating qualities. Whenever water is to be applied continuously to the surface, so as to be absorbed, as in the long tepid or half-bath, the sitz-bath, and for compresses, bandages and wet sheet packs, use soft water, if it can be procured—and more especially for drinking. Sea-bathing is peculiarly stimulating, tonic, and invigorating.

The temperature of water for ordinary bathing should be considerably below that of the body. The tem-perature of the blood varies but slightly from 98 de-grees Fahrenheit. A very feeble person may bathe in water at 70 degrees, but those who are more vigorous should use it colder; and the lower the temperature, the more sudden and powerful is the shock, and the more rapid and perfect the re-action. The immediate effect of cold water is to drive the blood from the part to which it is applied. The nerves, feeling the want of blood, as the element of vitality, and of warmth, which is the sensible expression of vitality, call it back. This is what is termed re-action. The blood returns, producing redness, a glowing warmth, and a feeling of vigour in the part. You may try this by merely dip-ping the hand in very cold water a few minutes; or you may try it on the whole surface of the body. In this way we strengthen the whole skin; we act upon the periphery of the whole system of the nerves of sensation; we quicken the action of millions of capillaries; we strengthen the circulation; we invigorate the whole body.

The effect of warm water, on the other hand, is to soften sensation, expand the capillaries, lower the tone, and enfeeble the action. Hot water, indeed, is stimulating, but its subsequent effect is debilitating. It is little used in water-cure, for this reason; but we sometimes resort to it in emergencies. For example, in congestion of the brain or lungs, we put the feet and legs into hot water, while we apply cold to the part affected. We also apply warm water to a part when we wish to backen a crisis, subdue irritation, diminish action, lessen certain secretions, as that of milk in the breasts, or diminish inflammation. The warm bath has also a soothing effect upon the nervous system, calms irritable nerves, and moderates convulsive action. Warm hip-baths and hot fomentations are used to allay uterine pains, and give relief in colic. But the very property by which warm water soothes makes it weakening, and it is to be avoided, except in emergencies.

Pain of the most violent kind, and even convulsions, are cured by the application of cold water; but it should be very cold and applied freely. In inflammations, fevers, and in all cases where the heat of the system is kept up, we may apply cold without fear. It is in cases of great exhaustion, internal congestion, and collapse, *without the strength to re-act*, that cold i dangerous. Even in these conditions, when applie quickly, and in a way to secure re-action, it is some-times of the greatest benefit.

The General Bath.—Every person should be washed all over in water, at least once every day of their lives. In infancy or age, at home or abroad, sick or well, there should be the daily ablution. Every square inch of skin on the whole body needs it, just as much as the face and hands; and it can be done, at a pinch, with a pint of water, with the hand, a wet towel, or a sponge. With two or three quarts of water, and a sponge or towel, you can have a glorious bath; begin by washing the head, an l then the entire body. End by a thorough rubbing with hands and towels, the coarser the better, and you have done your skin something like justice.

A more thorough and exciting bath may be taken by placing before the wash-stand a broad shallow pan or tub to stand in; then use the sponge as before, squeezing the water over the head or back of the neck and letting it flow down the body.

A towel bath is preferred by some to a sponge bath. Fold the towel lengthwise once, then across. Dip this quarto in the basin and wash face, head, and arms, stooping over the pan. Now step into it, dip the towel into the wash-basin, and wash down the chest, abdomen, and legs; open out the full length, dip, and saw down the back from head to knees; fold, and wash down in front, finishing with the feet; squat down on haunches and thoroughly wash the lower part of the body; stand up, and raising the wash-bowl to the chin, pour the water so as to run down over the whole body. Wipe thoroughly with a soft and then with a rough towel, combining vigorous exercise with a lively friction.

Some kind of a general bath should be taken on rising, except where the debility and consequent chilliness are too great, when it may be postponed to mid-forenoon. A bath is also always taken on coming out of either a wet sheet or blanket pack, or vapour, or hot air bath. The warmer a person is the better he can bear a full bath, and it is never better than when the body is covered with perspiration. The common notion about taking cold from a bath is quite unfounded. If a man thoroughly fatigued and over-heated, goes into cold water, and remains long, it may produce a severe and even fatal chill ; but a quick bath and good rubbing is always refreshing. In dry and feverish states of the system, a bath may be taken as often as it is agreeable, if every hour. When a fever patient is too feeble to stand up and be bathed, he may be washed, lying down, with a sponge or towel. In whatever manner taken, the bath is cooling, cleansing, and invigorating, though it may prove warming to a cold person, by exciting reaction, and increasing the vigour of the circulation.

The Dripping Sheet is a capital general bath, especially for invalids who require assistance. It can be had wherever there is a clean sheet and water enough to wet it. Let it just drip, throw it around the person to be bathed, and rub over it with the hands for half a minute or longer.

The Pouring-Bath.—One or two pails of water poured over the patient, who stands or crouches in a tub is also one of the best in use. There are few persons who cannot take one pail of cold water poured quickly over them, and followed by a brisk rubbing. The weakest persons bear such a bath, and feel the stronger for taking it.

The Plunge-Bath is any way of getting into the water all over, wetting the head first, as in all general baths. The common long baths are very good, but a tank of cold spring water four or five feet deep and large enough to swim in, is glorious. This bath, especially by all weak persons, should be taken quickly. Plunge in, and jump out again, dance about, and have a good rubbing. If you go into a river, or place large enough to swim, the exercise will enable you to stay in longer ; but even here, staying in too long produces exhaustion.

The Shower-Bath is often injurious, from the strong chill it produces, without exciting sufficient reaction. It is seldom used in water-cure.

The Half-Bath.—This is one of the most powerful

P

means of acting upon the whole system, reducing fever, removing local congestions, equalising the circulation, and controlling spasmodic action. The patient sits in a tub—a common bathing-tub is best—with the water four inches deep. He is then wet-rubbed all over with the hands of one or two, and water poured over him with a pail, from time to time, or dashed forcibly against him as the rubbing proceeds, in which the patient, if able, should assist. I have used this bath in severe congestive fever, with the water at 80 degrees, applying colder water to the head and chest, with great advantage. Priesnitz used this bath quite cold in many cases, and sometimes for four or five hours at a time, and with it he relieved severe congestions, ague, lockjaw, insanity, and cholera, even in the stage of collapse. The rubbing should be thorough, and made by relays of assistants, when it is long continued. When the patient comes out, let him be dry-rubbed and wrapped up in blankets—not packed, but well covered in bed.

The Sitz-Bath.—This admirable bath may be taken very well in a medium-sized washing-tub, but the ordinary hip-bath is more convenient. Fill it so that when the patient sits in it it will be half-full of water. It is well to begin with about 70 degrees in ordinary cases, and make it colder every day, until we come down to the common temperature of well or spring water. What I mean by 70 degrees, if you have no thermometer, is water "with the chill off," or moderately cool. Remove the clothing sufficiently, and sit in the water, from three to six inches deep, from five to fifteen minutes. You may aid the effect by rubbing the submerged surface with the hand. When you come out, dry and rub the parts with a towel; and if the water is cold, you will find the immersed skin nearly the colour of a boiled lobster. This tells what is going on in the capillary system. It is well for delicate persons to begin with cool water—water with the chill off, and use it colder every day until they can take it quite cold.

The cold sitz-bath relieves congestion of the brain, cures piles and constipation, dysentery, and is a sovereign remedy for weakness of the generative organs, falling of the womb, ovarian diseases, etc. It should be taken through pregnancy, and afterward until full recovery. Every such bath gives a strength that no one can conceive of, who has not tried it, or seen its beneficial operation.

The Douche.—This is a stream of water, of an inch or more in diameter, falling from ten to twenty feet. It is a very powerful application, bringing a great quantity of water rapidly to act upon a surface, and with considerable mechanical force. It must not be taken on the head, which must be first wet, but may fall upon the whole length of the spine, and on the chest and limbs, for from one to five minutes. It is a most powerful invigorator. It excites great capillary action, even to the dispersion of indolent tumours. Patients are so excited and toned up by this bath, that they are apt to take more than is prescribed to them.

An Ascending Douche, or fountain-bath, may be constructed with a rising stream of water, so as to act upon the lower part of the pelvis. It is excellent for piles, disease of the prostate, and seminal weaknesses in men, and for corresponding affections in women; and is an admirable remedy for all the irritations, inflammations, weaknesses, and morbid conditions of the lower bowel, womb, and generally of the pelvic viscera. The rising douche, or fountain-bath, may be found at most hydropathic establishments, but was not until now available in home or general practice. I have, however, recently invented a portable fountain-bath, or rising douche, which has several striking advantages. It can be used in the bed-room or dressing-room of the patient, supplied with fresh or salt water of any temperature, and its force is under perfect and instant control. It is furnished at a moderate price, and can be sent to any part of the world.

Head-baths, hand-baths, foot-baths, etc., are full or partial immersions of these parts in water. The head-bath is taken lying on the floor with the head resting in a basin of water; but a wet towel upon the head, renewed as required, is more convenient. When the feet and hands are habitually cold, they may be treated together, by dipping them in cold water a moment, then taking them out, and rubbing the feet with the hands, and repeating the process until both are warm.

The Vapour-Bath.—The steam or vapour-bath is not much used in water-cure, but where a quick and powerful action of the skin is desired, it is often useful. In severe colds, with a dry skin and chilly extremities, a single vapour-bath, followed by a good wash-down, sometimes effects a cure. Sit on a common cane-bottom chair, have blankets or a similar covering pinned around you, so as to leave your head free; place under the chair a tin vessel of water, over a spirit lamp. The water, to save time, may be first brought to the boiling point. For want of a proper lamp, the alcohol, or strong spirit of any kind, may be burnt in an open cup. Or, placing boiling water under the chair, the steam may be raised by putting in it hot irons, bricks, or stones. In a few moments the perspiration begins. It may go on for twenty minutes. Come out, and take a thorough cold bath. This must never be neglected. It is the only way in which the skin can be left in good condition.

The Lamp-bath is given in the same way, but with the lamp only, or burning spirits, without water. It is occasionally useful. but too debilitating for regular treatment.

The Wet Compress.—This is a napkin or towel, wrung out of cold water, folded into four or eight thicknesses, and laid upon the part affected. If it is an inflamed part we wish to cool, it may be left uncovered and often renewed. If, on the contrary, it is a torpid part, in which we wish to excite action, we cover the compress, and let it remain acting like a poultice. This last application is of great use in cases of indolent swellings, rheumatic joints, torpid livers, indurated spleens, weak stomachs, etc.

Fomentations are compresses wrung out of hot water; and to relieve pains, dissipate congestion, and lessen the action of the part.

The Wet Bandage.—This is an extension of the compress, and one of the most convenient and salutary applications in water-cure. As commonly worn, it is a towel, folded two or more thicknesses, so as to make a girdle ten inches wide. It is wrung out of cold water, and pinned around the loins so as to cover the lower part of the abdomen. It is a wonderful support, and strengthens better than body braces or supporters, which weaken the muscles they are intended to aid. The wet bandage should be worn during pregnancy, and in all cases of female weakness. It acts upon the great nervous centres of the abdominal and pelvic viscera. It may be worn night and day, and renewed as often as it gets dry or feels uncomfortable. If it cause chilly sensations, wear more covering or a dry bandage, flannel, or otherwise, over it.

Wet bandages are also worn around the middle, to strengthen the stomach, and excite the action of the liver—around the chest, in bronchial and pulmonary affections, to relieve the mucous membrane, by exciting the action of the skin—and around the throat, in either acute or chronic affections in that region.

The Wet Jacket, made of towelling or coarse linen, or cotton, without sleeves, and so as to cover the

whole chest with a tolerable fit, pinning over in front,
may be wrung out of cold water, and worn as a substi-
tute for the bandage. Wear clothing enough, night
and day, so as not to chill.

The Wet-Sheet Pack is a curative agent of astonishing efficacy. It consists of one or two comfortables,
three or four woollen blankets, and a linen or cotton
sheet.

Spread the blankets, which should be moderately
warm in cold weather, on the bed, with pillows at the
head under them. Take a sheet, large or small, thick
or thin, as the case requires ; wring it pretty close out
of cold water—spread it on the blankets. Let the
patient lie down at full length on the sheet, which
must be quickly folded around him. Then bring over
the first blanket, first one side and then the other,
drawing it closely around the neck, tucking it about
the feet, and making it snug all the way down. Do
the same with each blanket, making all comfortably
snug. The Germans put a small feather bed over
all, and tuck it in well ; but the comfortables, or any
common bed covering will answer the same purpose.
There must be covering enough, and the outer one
less pervious than blankets. See that the feet are well
wrapped up, and that the head is in a good position.
If the patient is feverish, the sheet may cover all but
the face. If inclined to be chilly, the sheet may only
come down to the ankles. Sometimes we begin by
letting the sheet come down only to the knees; sometimes by only putting a wet towel around under the
arms. These are partial wet-sheet packs.

In most cases, the sensations of the patient in the
pack are delightful after the first shock of the sheet.
In five minutes there is a glow all over the body; then
comes an indescribably calm, soothing feeling, from
the emollient effect of the wet sheet upon the skin, or
the nerves of sensation. All pain is relieved better

than by any opiate. Generally, in ten or fifteen minutes, the patient is in a calm, beautiful sleep. In an hour or less, he breaks out into a profuse perspiration. Now is the time to take him out, by undoing the coverings quickly, and as quickly giving him some kind of a full bath, a dripping sheet, a sponge-bath, a pouring-bath, or any kind of a quick thorough wash-down with cold water. A good wiping and rubbing with coarse towels and the bare hands, completes the operation.

In fevers the packs may be short and frequent, but in all chronic cases they should be long enough for a full action on the skin. Sensible perspiration may not come at first, and a general glow is sufficient.

There is no absolute time for a wet-sheet pack. One patient may be hot, restless, and even in a perspiration in half an hour; another may warm up slowly, and require to stay in two hours. When the pack is likely to be a long one, let the patient empty the bladder just before going in. In long packs, a urinal may also be put in, so as to be used without coming out.

For children, the blankets may be folded, and the sheets made of a proportional size. Infants a week old take the full wet-sheet packs (in a thin towel) with great advantage. In all the diseases of infancy, in the inflammation and irritation of teething, in pain of the bowels, in feverishness, it gives instant relief. In measles, chicken-pox, and scarlet fever, it cannot be too soon resorted to, nor scarcely too often repeated, except in delicate children, where packing in the wet sheet, after the fever is subdued, may be injurious. But for all febrile and eruptive diseases, it is the sovereign remedy, and brings out these eruptions in the most wonderful manner. The most cross, sickliest baby generally goes to sleep in five minutes after being put in the pack.

The Sweating Blanket Pack is the same process, but without the wet sheet. Pack the patient in blankets thoroughly, and let him stay in until he sweats. If not too tired, he may sweat half an hour; then take him out, and give him a bath.

The blanket pack may also be given just long enough to accumulate heat, so that the patient may take a cold bath with advantage. The sweating pack is used where we wish to purify the system rapidly by the action of the skin, and where we wish to excite this organ. It may be used alternately with the wet-sheet in skin diseases, as salt rheum, in chronic rheumatism, in asthma and bronchitis, and in all torpid and poisoned conditions. Patients full of quinine, calomel, opium, or tobacco, if they can bear this process, find it a rapid means of cure. In affections of the throat, the blanket pack often proves successful, alternating with other methods, especially with the wet-sheet pack. When patients are chilling, a hot bottle may be placed at the feet; but artificial heat is to be used with caution.

I have already spoken of injections to the rectum and vagina. The latter should be cool or cold, and taken with a syringe that will hold eight or ten ounces, with a tube, the globular end of which is pierced with several small holes. By this means cold water may be thrown forcibly upon the uterus. These injections, to the amount of two quarts at a time, may be taken several times a-day, and no woman should be without the means of taking them. They remedy, and if persevered in, with other right habits, cure every weakness and disease of the female sexual organs. I have adopted injection and irrigation tubes to my Portable Fountain Bath, so that they can be taken with great facility.

Old persons, delicate women, and feeble children must be treated with care, and it is better, to be safe, to make the water a few degrees warmer, than to do mischief. There is danger in certain persons of producing congestion of the lungs, by giving too cold sitz or other baths. In giving packs, the water in which the sheet is wet should be quite cold, but we may lessen the size of the sheet, and wring it close. The baths which follow a pack must also be cold, but may be very quickly given. But in sitz-baths, rubbing-baths, rising douche, and injections, the water may be used with the chill off, especially at beginning.

It is not necessary to suspend treatment during menstruation. Time is needlessly lost, and it is at this time that women most need treatment. Wear the bandage, take sitz-baths, and use the vagina syringe the same as usual.

All sheets, bandages, compresses, etc., used in water cure must be washed every day, and often boiled, or they are made very filthy by the impurities which come from the skin. If the same cloths are used without washing, these matters are re-absorbed.

Every mother should have a small syringe, holding two or three ounces, to give injections to her infants. Some children have torpid bowels until they are three months old. Much medicine and misery may be saved by the use of injections.

A water emetic should be taken whenever there is more gastric irritation from matter in the stomach than merely drinking a glass of water will quell. Drink as much lukewarm water as you can swallow, then tickle the fauces with your finger or the feather end of a quill.

No cold bath, pack, or any process requiring reaction, should be taken within half an hour before or two hours after a meal. When the blood and nervous power are in the skin they cannot be secreting gastric juice for the stomach, nor *vice versa*. We cannot act powerfully with two great organs at the same time, and the blood and vitality go where there is the loudest call. Eat a hearty meal, and then take violent exercise,

or exert great mental effort, or take a cold bath, and
you produce a chill, or, perhaps, vomiting—perhaps a
long fit of indigestion.

Bathing is exercise. If any other be taken, let it be
vigorous and brief before and after.

GENERAL DIRECTIONS:

The mind of the patient should be free from all care,
trouble, anxiety, sorrow, or irritation. Avoid gloomy
conversation and thought. Shun repulsive occupation
and unpleasant society.

Labour or exercise so as to produce moderate fatigue,
but not exhaustion. No greater fatigue should be
incurred than a night's rest will remove. Exercise in
the open air, and as many muscles as you can. If
walking is too exhausting, ride on horseback or in a
carriage. If not able to take exercise, be rubbed freely
over the whole body.

Be much in the open air, and have all your rooms
well ventilated. Windows should be open at top and
bottom, with no impediment from shades and curtains.
Breathe pure, fresh air, night and day. Have your
rooms light as well as airy. Exposure of the whole
body to air and light, even the direct rays of the sun,
when not too powerful, is a potent means of cure.

The dress must be light, loose, clean, and comfortable in regard to temperature. No article must be
worn at night that is worn by day; and all clothing,
for person or bed, should be thoroughly aired, daily
and nightly. Keep the body warm with sufficient
underclothing — under-jackets and drawers. Many
people, and especially delicate women, suffer from
continual chilliness. Underclothing should be often
changed—the cleaner the better.

Sleep on a mattress of hair, wool, straw, etc.; not
on feathers. The covering should be very clean,
thoroughly aired daily, light, porous, warm, but not

too warm. A hot water bottle is better than cold feet, but it should be removed as soon as possible.

A water-cure diet excludes all fat, greasy, oily substances, except a small quantity of oil or good butter; all smoked or very salt meats and fish, pickles and preserves; all pork, lard, sausages, mince pies, geese, ducks, veal, eels, and all oily fish, and all high-seasoned made-dishes, gravies, sauces, rich cake or pastry, spices, or condiments, except a moderate use of vinegar, salt, and sugar, honey, or molasses. Tea, coffee, spirits, tobacco, and all medicinal drugs, are strictly prohibited.

Abundant and healthful nutriment may be found in the following articles :—

Farinacea.—Wheat, unbolted, as bread or porridge; oatmeal porridge, or gruel; rye bread, Indian corn bread, hominy, etc. ; rice, tapioca, sago, arrowroot, etc.

Fruit.—Apples, peaches, pears, strawberries, grapes, whortleberries, blackberries, plums, bananas, melons, oranges, figs, dates. In winter, stewed apples, peaches, prunes, etc.

Vegetables.—Potatoes, common and sweet, green peas, shell and string beans, turnips, beets, broccoli, cabbage, onions, carrots, parsnips, spinach, spring greens, etc.

Animalised Substances.—Milk, cream, butter, mild and tender cheese ; eggs—soft-boiled, poached, scrambled, or made in a custard or omelette—and, in all cases, slightly cooked, etc.

Fish.—Scale fish, fresh and in their season. Oysters, do., raw or cooked rare.

Flesh.—Lean mutton, beef, venison, chicken, turkey, wild fowl of a similar character. White meats are preferable to dark.

The best cures are made upon a simple vegetable diet. When persons *will* eat animal food, the above varieties are least hurtful.

A strict diet consists of a few of the best articles of farinacea and fruit, with a little milk, in all not exceeding six ounces of *nutriment* a-day. *A moderate diet* may include a greater variety of articles, and ten ounces of nutriment. *A full diet*, suitable to a condition of health, may vary from twelve to sixteen ounces of nutriment a-day. Of course the water which forms so large a portion of fruits and vegetables is not reckoned as nutriment.

Eat slowly, masticate thoroughly, and be sure that a single ounce more than the stomach can readily digest, without uneasiness, acts as an irritant, and exhausts vitality. Rest mind and body after every meal. Take no bath for half an hour before, or two hours after eating. Eat at regular intervals. When more than two meals a-day are taken, let the last meal be lightest; and no invalid should eat later than four P.M., or six hours before retiring to rest. If in pain, or wearied, or without an appetite, *fast*. Fatigue, before eating, may hinder digestion, as may labour, excitement, or any exhausting process after it.

No food should be put in the mouth hot, and none should be *swallowed* cold; that will be prevented by a good mastication.

Milk being classed as food, the only drink should be pure, soft water. Where the spring water is hard, filtered or clean rain water is better. The quantity drank may be in proportion to thirst and exercise, but even pure, soft water may be taken to excess. If drinking chills, sip slowly, and in small quantities at a time.

Where the capital stock of *vitality* has been reduced, it must be husbanded with care. Amative excitement and indulgence, of whatever kind, and under whatever circumstances, must be carefully avoided. More vitality may be lost in one moment, than can be gained by weeks of persevering treatment. In the young of both sexes, the debilitated, those labouring under chronic disease, in female weaknesses, and during gestation and lactation, there should be no excitement of the roductive system. Parents cannot too carefully

guard their children against the health and life-destroy-
ing abuses of this function, from which the period of
infancy is not always exempt.

It will be evident that in the water-cure processes
we act chiefly upon the surface of the body. This
surface comprises about fifteen square feet. It contains millions of sudoriferous or sweat-making glands,
and a vast number of sebaceous or oil-secreting. It
contains an immense capillary reticulation, and a
wonderful expansion of nerves, both organic and sensational. In acting upon the skin, we have the means
of influencing the whole system as we can in no other
manner. We can weaken or strengthen, enliven or
depress, bring the blood to the surface or drive it back
upon the viscera.

By exciting the action of the skin, we rapidly free
the system of its impurities, and relieve, rest, and
invigorate the internal organs. An oppression of the
lungs is relieved almost instantly by opening the pores,
and increasing the action of the skin; a diarrhœa is
quickly cured by making the skin throw off the matter
which is coming from the mucous membrane. Profuse expectorations from chronic bronchitis are rapidly
diminished in this way, and attacks of asthma relieved
and cured.

The changes of nutrition, waste, and excretion are
so much quickened in water-cure, that Liebig, who
examined it carefully at Graefenburg, says in a letter
to Sir Charles Scudamore, that as great a change is
often effected in six weeks as would be accomplished
in three years without it. The system is therefore
freed from its old diseased matter, and built up with
new materials with wonderful rapidity. It is rather
important, then, that the new matter of nutrition
should be of the purest quality.

The quantity and quality of morbid matter thrown
from the skin, the lungs, the kidneys, and the bowels,

during a course of water-cure, is sometimes astonishing, even to those best acquainted with its efficacy. The bath-room is filled with dense vapour by the active skin; and we can smell opium, tobacco, mercury, and other drugs which may have been taken years before. The blankets used in packing require to be thoroughly aired every day. I have been poisoned by inhaling this diseased matter, and I was once inoculated with it, by handling a sheet in which a patient had been packed. Patients have collected globules of mercury which came out under their wet bandages, though they had taken none for years. Bandages and sheets are often stained by matters which come from the skin, and they are at times so corroded as to fall in pieces. It is not uncommon to have them stiff with glutinous exudations.

But at times, and especially when packing and bandaging are not enough attended to, these out-pourings of morbid matter are of a more violent and painful character. This is what is called *crisis*. There is a sudden breaking up of morbid matter, which comes away in a mass, sometimes by a flood of thick or gravelly urine; sometimes by a violent sweating which lasts for days; sometimes by vomiting; often by a diarrhoea which will last for a week and carry off an unaccountable quantity of matter; very commonly by an eruption on the skin, which may come out over the whole surface, but more likely under the compresses and bandages, or over the seat of disease; or, lastly—and this is the severest form of crisis—the patient may have crops of boils over the whole body. I have known forty at a time. They are unpleasant, but bring a wonderful relief. As they pour out matter, the internal organs are left free from it, and I have seen a troublesome cough, with profuse expectoration, quite cured by the appearance of a crop of boils over the chest, which threw off matter precisely like that which had been expectorated. All these facts go strongly to confirm Francke's theory of the "sliming up" of morbid matter, until some action is set up by nature, or by water-cure processes, in aid of nature, to set it free. When the system is filled with this matter, though we may seem to be in health, it is always oppressing us; and a large portion of our strength is expended in guarding it; the least disturbance, as cold or fatigue, sets free a portion of it; it always tends to any exhausted or weakened part; it finds its way into wounds; it keeps up ulcerations; it is liable to oppress the brain by tuberculous gatherings, or cause consumption of the lungs, or disease of the mesenteric glands, or other fatal disorders.

In the scientific and judicious practice of the water-cure, this matter is carried out of the system, generally without any violent crisis. A pure nutrition supplies the place of the bad matter removed, and the whole organism is built up afresh. When crisis occurs, the patient is to fast, rest, and moderate his treatment. Use the water a little less cold; in sweating, wash often; in diarrhœa, fast and take frequent injections; in eruptions and boils, take wet-sheet packs.

There are diseased conditions which no treatment can cure, or long relieve. When a vital organ has been destroyed, or made permanently useless, the patient must sink. When vitality has been so exhausted by any cause that the process of purification cannot be carried on, the poor body must clog up and perish. When a certain amount of disease has settled upon the brain or its membranes, or the spinal cord; when the lungs are solidified or disorganised, so as to prevent the uses of respiration; when the liver can no longer perform its function; when digestion is destroyed; when the mesenteric glands are solidified or tuberculated, clogged up with diseased matters; when the kidneys fail; when the heart is disorganised; when the organic nervous system can no longer give vigour to the capillary system, and carry on the processes of nutrition and secretion, then comes the inevitable Death. A wise use of the directions given in this book will aid nature in doing all possibilities; but some diseases, or conditions of disease, are inevitably fatal.

Although I say little of the use of medicines, believing that most of the drugs used of late years in Allopathic medication do more evil than good, I have no wish to utterly condemn them. There is evident use, in many cases, in a quick, active emetic. One may do much worse than take a dose of castor-oil, or epsom salts, or many of the aperient mineral waters, in any special need; but it is not well to be in the habit of using any cathartic medicine whatever. So of stimulants. One may take wine or spirits in an emergency with benefit—but the habit of resorting to them is weakening and dangerous. The same with opiates and all anesthetic agents. Chloroform has been fatal to many. Ether is much less dangerous. The nitrous oxide gas, now so much used in dental operations, is comparatively safe, but has not been so in all cases. Chloral, the new opiate, is very seductive, and dangerous to use habitually. Pure health needs no stimulation or medication.

Genuine Homœopathy is assuredly harmless; and there is abundant testimony to the efficacy of many homœopathic medicines, as of belladonna in throat diseases and scarlatina. Many water-cure physicians give the proper homœopathic remedies. And the experience, perhaps we may say the instincts, of mankind testify to the benefit, in a multitude of cases, of simple vegetable medicines, roots and herbs, and the herb teas, made of roots, leaves, and flowers, so largely used in France, and more or less among all civilised and savage nations.

The Turkish Bath, I need hardly say, is, in the cases to which it is adapted, and with those to whom it can be adapted, a rapid and powerful mode of purification and invigoration.

CHAPTER XVII.

DISEASES AND TREATMENT.

MEDICAL systems vary in the nomenclature and classification of diseases. They are divided into local and general, organic and functional. In medical books we have enumerated—

Diseases of Periods—infancy, manhood, old age.

Diseases of Sex—as those peculiar to men and women.

Diseases of Regions—as of the head, chest, abdomen, pelvis.

Diseases of Condition or Callings—as of the rich, the poor, professional men, literary men, artists, manufacturers, labourers, etc.

Diseases of Function—as of digestion, circulation, respiration, secretion, innervation, generation, gestation, locomotion, etc.

Diseases of Tissues—as of the skin, mucous and serous membranes, vascular, nervous, fibrous, osseous tissues, etc.

Diseases of Organs—as the eye, ear, throat, brain, lungs, stomach, liver, kidneys, uterus, etc., etc.

In the system of Dr. Farr, adopted by the Registrar-General, diseases are divided into four classes, each including nerval orders. Under Class I.—*Zymotic Diseases* (*zymé*, a ferment,) are included epidemic, endemic, and contagious diseases, and those caused

by specific poisons, and food or want of food. The
four orders are 1.—*Miasmatic Diseases* (tainted), as
small-pox, measles, scarlet fever, diphtheria, typhus
and typhoid fevers, cholera, ague, etc. Order 2.
Enthetic Diseases (implanted), as syphilis, gonorrhœa,
glanders, hydrophobia, malignant pustule, etc. Order
3. *Dietic Diseases*, as famine-fever, scurvy, purpura,
rickets, delirium tremens, and all the effects of stimulants and narcotics. Order 4. *Parasitic Diseases*, as
itch, worms, ring-worm, scald-head, etc.

Class II.—*Constitutional Diseases*, containing two
orders. 1. *Diathetic Diseases*, as gout, anemia, cancer,
etc. ; and 2. *Tubercular Diseases*, as scrofula, phthisis
(tubercular consumption), mesenteric disease, etc.
These are, for the most part, hereditary.

Class III.—*Local Diseases*, contains, order 1.
Diseases of the Brain or Nervous System, as apoplexy,
paralysis, epilepsy, chorea (St. Vitus' dance), hysteria,
mania, etc. 2. *Diseases of the Heart and Blood-
Vessels*. 3. *Lung Diseases*, as bronchitis, pneumonia,
pleurisy, asthma, etc. 4. *Diseases of the Digestive
System*, as inflammations of the stomach or intestines,
jaundice, etc. ; and orders 5, 6, and 7 are diseases of
the kidneys, generative organs, bones, muscles, and
skin. Class IV. includes *Developmental Diseases*. 1.
In children, as malformations, idiocy, teething; 2.
Of women, relating to menstruation and childbirth;
3. Of old age; 4. Of nutrition, as atrophy, debility, etc.

In examining the patient to ascertain the nature of
the disease, the points necessary for the physician to
know are the age; sex; condition, bodily, mental,
and social; relations, married or single, children, etc. ;
parentage, and the probabilities of hereditary predispositions; past history of patient, diseases and
medication; regularity of certain functions, as menstruation or defæcation; the amative function, strong
or weak, exercised or not solitarily or socially, and,

in either case, to what extent; present condition; pain; tenderness; derangement of action, and what kind; pulse; respiration; state of mind and temper; strength; disposition to exercise, state of the skin, tongue, teeth, hair, senses.

There are nervous affections dependent upon exhaustion, that are difficult to locate or find a name for; flying pains which change about from one part to another; the feelings usually termed hysterical, and states of depression and general weakness, which come from bodily, or mental, or spiritual exhaustion. But in most cases, we are able to locate a disease in the head, the chest, the abdomen, the pelvis, the bones, the joints, the muscles, the nerves, the blood-vessels, the glands, the membranes, or the skin. We pursue the investigation until the complaint is cornered. We find where it is not, and then narrow it down to where it is. In a personal examination, the physician, taking in with one glance twenty other particulars, as they are disclosed by the appearance, complexion, weight, motions, attitudes, and tones of the patient, may ask first of all, "Where is the pain?" Another will sit down more patiently, and say, "What is the story?"

There are certain signs of diseases which are worthy of special attention.

A bad smelling breath is a sign of foul or decaying teeth, indigestion, or constipation.

Early decay of teeth is a sign of hereditary weakness, early exhaustion, or chronic dyspepsia.

A tongue creased, and cut into deep furrows, is a sign of dyspepsia.

Light hair, fair complexion, and a thick upper lip, are signs of scrofula.

A dry, hard skin, and cold extremities, are signs of nervous exhaustion. Hollow eyes, dark circles around them, flabbiness, and emaciation, are all signs of exhausting causes of disease. A moist, clammy skin is sometimes found in dyspepsia.

A pulse steadily above a hundred a minute in an adult, indicates high general fever, or severe internal inflammation. If in a chronic case, and combined with regularly progressive emaciation, it indicates a dangerous and probably fatal disease of some vital organ.

An unnaturally slow pulse, a feeble pulse, and an intermitting pulse, are signs of great nervous exhaustion. A small pulse with rigors, is a sign of internal congestion, or what is the same thing, a want of action in the external capillaries.

Paralysis, insensibility, with regular and rather slow pulse, and deep breathing, show compression of the brain from injury or apoplexy.

Delirium is a sign of cerebral congestion without effusion.

Other signs of disease will be noted as we come to the symptoms which characterise those we are about to describe, for the aggregate of symptoms is the real description of a disease.

There are diseases of the mind, and affections or sentiments, as well as of the bodily organs.

Home Sickness is a common, and sometimes a fatal disease. Its cause is simply a removal from home. The more striking the change, the severer the malady. A Swiss who leaves his Alps, an Arab taken from his desert, and a Greenlander from his icebergs, all suffer from the pangs of this disease. It is marked by pining, melancholy, sighing, weeping, depression, and death. The cure is to return home ; if this is impracticable, some other passion should be excited, as ambition or love.

Love Sickness is like the last, but more common, and often more severe. A disappointment in love sometimes crushes and kills. The patient may-die suddenly of a broken heart, or gradually pine away. Its symptoms are like those of home sickness, but more tender and pitiful. Sometimes the intellect is affected with a temporary or permanent derangement. It is the most frequent cause of suicide.

Union with the object beloved is a cure, if it comes in season; a cure is also often happily effected by transferring the affection to another object. Other passions also are a relief, and any employment of the mind which interests or gives vivid pleasure. Travel, art, reading, occupation, benevolence, and religion, are all useful.

Religion, or the combined passions of faith, hope, reverence, and conscientiousness, is often in a state of disease. We have no mad-house without its religious maniacs. As this is a more complex sentiment, its modes of disease are more varied. Great efforts are made in revivals, camp-meetings, and on many other occasions to excite this feeling; and we often see its morbid manifestations. These are, at times, reflected upon the body, producing strange convulsions, swoonings, paroxysms and ecstasies. In its mild form it is enthusiasm; in its severe, fanaticism; in its repulsive, it is bigotry. This disease is often acute, and commonly epidemic. It is also clearly contagious.

Jealousy is a very bad and a very prevalent passional disease, and few diseases cause more anguish to the sufferer, or more discomfort to others. It is often treated as a wickedness—we may call it so, if we please, but it is a disease. A wickedness, properly speaking, is a voluntary thing. Jealousy is involuntary. It is sudden or gradual, violent or mild, acute or chronic. It has its own internal, pre-disposing, cause; but the external exciting cause may be either real or imaginary. It is a morbid manifestation of love, combined with distrust, fear, and spiritual poverty.

How shall we cure jealousy? It has been argued

against by the philosophers, and ridiculed by the wits of all ages. It disorders the mind, sours the temper, affects the appetite and digestion, seems to interfere with the bilious secretion, and gives a dull, hard pain around the heart. It leads oftener than any other passional disease to suicide and murder.

In passional diseases, we must adopt appropriate modes of treatment. Many are cured by friendship, or ambition, or love. Many are benefited by music, by books, by society. I have known a severe and long-continued fit of mental depression to be cured by a single tune. A world of new life may come into the soul from a beautiful picture, or a beautiful woman.

As a general rule, the best way to keep a healthy mind, is to give it a healthy body for its basis, so the best guarantee for spiritual health, is to preserve the health, the combined animal and organic systems.

I will endeavour to give such an account of diseases and treatment as the general reader can understand, and may find practically useful. I begin with some general diseases, and follow with diseases of systems, organs, etc.

Fever is the name given to a general and somewhat violent effort of the system to free itself from the matter of disease. Fevers are characterised by pain, heat, excitement of the circulating system, over-action of the organic, and consequent prostration of the locomotive.

The causes of fever are too great quantity or bad quality of food, want of cleanliness, bad air, poisonings of many kinds, with so much exhaustion, that the system cannot rid herself of their effects without a special effort. The immediate cause of an attack of fever may be chill, fatigue, worry, or any unusual cause of disturbance or exhaustion.

Fever begins, generally, with a chill or rigor, followed by pain in the head, back, and limbs, weakness, heat of the surface, throbbing of the arteries, loss of appetite, constipation; there is great thirst, quick pulse, hurried breathing; it terminates with more or less violent critical action, generally of the skin, in profuse sweatings, often with copious discharges from the kidneys and bowels.

The action in fever may be concentrated upon some particular portion of the system. If the disease is chiefly local, it is called inflammation, and the fever is considered sympathetic or symptomatic; but if there is much general disturbance, we speak of brain fever, lung fever, gastric fever, etc.

Intermittent Fever—chills and fever—fever and ague is one of the simplest and best defined forms of this disease. It begins with a chill, or rigor, which may last from half an hour to two or three hours; be mild or severe, with a shivering of the whole body, and a feeling of coldness which no fire can warm. The external capillaries collapse, and the blood is thrown upon the internal organs. The second stage is that of fever, with pain, throbbing, heat, thirst. This lasts an hour or two, and is followed by a crisis of perspiration. The attack is repeated on the next day but one, the third, or even the fourth day.

Cause.—Malaria, acting upon a system too weak to resist, or free itself in any other manner.

Effects.—This disease is not generally considered dangerous, but it is sometimes fatal to a weak and exhausted person. In such cases the chill may produce general collapse and coma, from which there is no reaction. As usually treated by quinine, arsenic, piperine, and other violent or insidious poisons, the cause of disease and the remedies both remain in the system, producing various chronic diseases.

Treatment.—As in all cases, we must aid nature in her efforts, keep them within safe limits, and as far as possible invigorate and purify. If practicable, the patient should remove from a malarious region. This alone is often sufficient for a cure. But if we must labour under the disadvantage of curing the disease, while subject to its cause, we must do the best we can.

The chill may be broken by a very cold pouring bath and rubbing, or by the half-bath. This produces a more rapid re-action. After the cold bath and rubbing, the patient may be enveloped in blankets. He may drink water freely, but not too cold. When the fever comes on, either give a succession of dripping sheets, or a wet-sheet pack. I prefer the latter. When the patient has sweated half an hour, give him a pouring-bath or dripping sheet; place him in a clean, cool bed, and let him rest.

But in whatever way he passes through the attack, the treatment must be kept up in the intervals. Give one or two wet-sheet packs on each well day. Every thorough pack is an artificial fit of chills and fever. When you go into the sheet, you have the cold stage; you re-act, heat accumulates, and you have the hot, or fever stage, and then comes the final stage of perspiration. This is nature's mode of cure. Every pack expels so much disease. By giving a rapid succession of packs, you may cure any ordinary case in from one to three weeks.

When the stomach is disordered, give tepid water emetics, and do not fail to move the bowels with daily injections.

Diet.—The less the patient eats the better, and the less he exercises or works, if he takes full treatment. The whole force of the system should be used to expel the disease.

Bilious Remittent Fever is, I believe, caused by the malaria of intermittent, combined with other malaria and personal causes of disease. It is a fever of remissions and exacerbations; but there is no entire freedom from its symptoms, as in fever and ague.

It commences with or without a chill; followed by

languor, weariness, uneasiness of stomach, pains in head, back, and limbs; then a hot, dry skin; full, bounding pulse, abrupt and frequent; restlessness, vomiting, thirst; tongue turns from white to yellow or brown; bowels constipated; stools green and acrid; severe stage lasts twelve to eighteen hours. This period usually comes on a little before noon. As the disease goes on, the vomiting becomes more frequent; there is heat and tenderness at the epigastrium, intolerable headache, and intolerance of light. The tongue becomes black, dries and cracks; respiration difficult; pulse sinks; prostration; twitchings of the muscles; death from seven to thirteen days. Often it sinks into a low stage, and lasts twenty or thirty days.

In Malignant Remittent, a severe form, or occurring in more poisoned and exhausted constitutions, the skin is cold and clammy; countenance pale, livid, and shrunk; pulse frequent and fluttering; stupor, or low delirium; syncope. Sometimes fatal in two or three days.

Effects.—As usually treated by bleeding and enormous doses of calomel and quinine, this disease is followed by jaundice, dyspepsia, enlargements of liver, spleen, etc., dropsy, consumption.

Treatment.—Cold water is the only reliable remedy. Even Professor Dickson, an allopath, says, "its remedial value cannot be exaggerated." Called to a severe case, I should try to give the patient a *cool* half-bath of twenty minutes' duration, with *cold* water to the head. If the stomach were disturbed, a water emetic. Then a thorough injection. As the fever came on again, a wet-sheet pack, as thorough as needed, and repeated as often. Cool water to drink, cool injections to the bowels, cold compresses upon the head, the wet-sheet pack, frequent, according to the violence of the fever; these are our means of cure, and carefully adapted to the necessities of each case, and the strength of each patient, they are sufficient to cure every curable case.

Diet.—Water, until the disease is conquered, then toast-water for a few days, and, very carefully, and in the smallest quantities, ripe fruit and farinaceous food. An indulgence in the cravings of the appetite, during recovery, is very dangerous. The stomach and bowels are so weak and irritable, that a single improper meal may be followed by fatal consequences.

Simple Continued Fever.—This name is given to a fever arising from the ordinary causes, and having no peculiar local determination. It often begins with chill, then pain, languor, and feverishness. It may be slight and brief, or severe and long continued, accord-ing to the amount of impurity, and the power of the system to expel it. If there is little matter of disease, and much vital energy, the fever will neither be long nor violent. If much disease and much energy, it will be violent, but short. It may also be a mild, slow fever, or a low and protracted one. In this case we call it typhus, and it may become malignant and contagious.

The Treatment.—Most fevers terminate in health. The diseasing matter is burned up and expelled, and the freed organism goes on with its functions. But we can guide and hasten this process. In all fevers, as in all diseases, we must surround the patient with the con-ditions of health. He must have pure air, cleanliness, and quiet; soft water to drink, *ad libitum;* the stomach should be thoroughly cleansed at the beginning, and the bowels washed clean at least once a day by a full injection. If the matter is acrid, twice a day is better. Let the whole skin be thoroughly washed at first with soap and tepid water. Use the wet-sheet pack as often and as long as the patient requires. If the fever is high, the packs may be short and more frequent. Sponging the whole surface, at intervals between the packs, is pleasant and useful. Fever is a fire, it is said, which we must put out. Not so; it is only an increase of a fire which is always burning. We must regulate this fire, and aid it in doing its work; and the more we wash away, the less there will be to burn.

Diet.—No fever patient has any business with food. Gruels and toast-water, rice-water, barley-water, broths, and all the slops of the sick room must be left out of it. A little lemonade is all that is allowable; and pure water is better than this. There is not the least danger in any sick person going a few days, and in the early stages of fever, without food. When the fever is gone, begin to eat with caution, and eat and live, in all respects, so as not to have another fever.

Typhus Fever of the mild kind, commonly called nervous fever, appears to be only simple fever with great nervous exhaustion. It is a fever of low type and slow progress; the determination to the skin is manifested in eruptions—minute, rose-coloured, chiefly about the chest. Later, eruptions like flea-bites are seen. In bad cases, toward the end of the second week, the patient sinks into great weakness, with tremors, picking of the bed-clothes, rapid pulse, red, dry tongue, dark mucous matter around the teeth, gloom and anxiety, low delirium, coma, brief convulsions, death.

The severer form of typhus, called *Putrid Fever*, *Jail Fever*, *Ship Fever*, is epidemic and contagious. It is marked by alternations of heat and cold; hot, dry, harsh skin; distress; face turgid and dark, red flush, eyes heavy and red; severe headache; pulse small, hard, tense, frequent, irregular; tongue coated with brown or yellowish fur; nausea and retching; bowels torpid. In three or four days the tongue becomes clean, dark, red, smooth, dry, cracked; sordes around teeth; pulse small and rapid; hurried respiration, or slow and laboured; foetid breath; eruption on the skin:

hemorrhages, and death, from the fifth to the thirtieth day.

Treatment.—If anything can save a patient in this form of the disease, it is the wet-sheet pack, combining invigoration and purification. Its effects seem more like miracles than the natural results of so simple a cause. But it does nearly all we wish to do. Water drinking, water injections, and the wet-sheet pack, followed by the full-bath, will cure ninety-nine cases in a hundred, even of the worst forms of this pestilential disorder. In the Franco-German war of 1870, the German troops attacked with Camp Typhus were treated with daily cold baths, and eighty per cent. recovered.

In all cases of fever, or other disease, accompanied with great muscular debility, the patient must be handled, and not made to exert himself. It may be necessary to give him all baths lying down. A large sponge is very convenient for this purpose. The German soldiers were taken up on their sheets by the four corners, and laid down into a bath tub; then, as soon as well cooled, lifted upon their cots, and wrapped in blankets.

Yellow Fever is classed as a continued fever; malarious and contagious. It requires prompt, thorough treatment, much the same as the bilious remittent.

Catarrhal Fever is the name given to influenza or common cold. Rest, warmth, and the wet-sheet pack are the best treatment. Even a cold bath, followed by a good rubbing, may cure. A full action of the skin by the vapour-bath, warm bath, Turkish bath, or blanket-pack, followed in either case by a cold bath, may be sufficient. The more morbid matter there is laid up in the system, the more severe are its disturbances. When this matter falls upon the nerves and the muscular system, we have painful rheumatisms. Stuffing a cold is a bad way to cure it. It may cure, as quinine cures ague, but only by making a morbid diversion, or inducing a different diseased action. Starve a cold, because a cold is a mild fever ; so that even the old saw is authority for this practice.

Symptomatic or Hectic Fever accompanies wounds and local inflammations. We are familiar with it in consumptive diseases. The whole system becomes disturbed from the local disturbance, or the action set up for the relief of one organ necessarily pervades the whole body. In this fever which is intermittent, recurring once or twice a-day, there is a quick pulse, a flush of the face, a bright, suffused eye, heat of the skin, and thirst. It is followed by profuse sweatings. Too much food excites this feverish action.

A sponge-bath, or the dripping sheet, used at the access of the fever, and again after the sweating has commenced, does much to control it.

Night sweats disappear in many cases when the skin is invigorated with daily bathing.

Scarlatina.—This contagious disease, an epidemic of bad air and uncleanly conditions, commences with symptoms like those of simple fever, but with determinations to the mucous membranes, and especially the throat. These are relieved, the second, the third, or fourth day by an eruption on the skin, consisting of small, isolated pimples, first pale red, then scarlet ; they enlarge, run together, and form large patches ; last seven to nine days, and disappear with a peeling off of the cuticle. The danger in this disease is, of its whole force being thrown upon the throat or the membranes of the brain. In weakly children, in the scrofulous, and in those exposed to unhealthy conditions, it is very fatal. Healthy children, living in healthy conditions, either entirely escape it, or are carried through it easily and rapidly by packing and bathing, so as to promote the full action of the skin and other treatment as in simple fever.

Measles—contagious, and usually occurs but once. It is characterised by an eruption of semi-lunar spots of vermillion red, separated by angular, colourless intervals. They begin at the roots of the hair, and travel gradually down over the body. The eyes are apt to be affected, and later, the lungs; sometimes the bowels. Where the skin is inactive, these internal affections are apt to be severe.

This disease is liable to be confounded with scarlatina; but this is of no consequence, as the treatment is the same. In both, the patient must fast, drink water, have water injections, and be packed twice a-day, or oftener, with spongings or pouring-baths. In Mrs. Nichols' "Woman's Work in Water Cure and Sanitary Education," she gives a case of measles, in which an infant had been seven days sleepless, with no eruption, and given up to die. It was wrapped in a wet-sheet pack. In ten minutes it was asleep; in half an hour, when taken out and bathed, the eruption covered the whole skin, and in two days it was out of danger. I have seen other cases saved by water, which were considered past all remedy. These diseases require prompt, bold treatment. The water must be cold, so as to insure a sufficient shock and a vigorous re-action.

The Small-Pox begins like a common fever, with chill, pains, gastric irritation, etc. In two or three days small red pimples appear on the neck, face, chest, and over the body. As they enlarge, they become white in the centre. In confluent small-pox, the pustules flatten and run together. The pustules dry up to scabs on the ninth to the eleventh day, and fall off from the fifteenth to the twentieth. Small-pox is highly contagious, and rages in unhealthy communities as a fatal epidemic. It was for a time supposed that vaccination was a safe-guard, but recent experience has shown that it does not prevent the disease, and that it is not seldom a means of communicating other diseases.

Small-pox owes its virulence to uncleanly habits and the eating of flesh. Vegetarians of pure lives and healthy constitutions are in no danger from it, and some will not take it by inoculation.

The treatment is the same as for any fever of the same intensity; protecting the skin by frequent packing, laying wet cloths upon it, and keeping out the light, as an additional safeguard against the pitting. It is seldom that a perceptible mark is left in judicious water-cure treatment.

Hooping or Whooping Cough, is of the same nature as the eruptive diseases of the skin. The dreadful cough is caused by the disease being determined to the mucous membrane. It has often been cured in ι week by abstinence, thorough wet-sheet packing, and the wet bandage around the chest.

The slighter infantile and eruptive fevers are to be treated on the same principles. Whenever a child is feverish, from any cause, there are certain things to be done. It must not eat nor nurse but very little; it may drink cold water, as much as it likes; its bowels must be moved, if they require it, by injections; and it must either be well bathed in cold water, or have a wet bandage around it, or be packed in a wet-sheet pack, or all three, if the symptoms require it. And in all cases observe that the amount of treatment is to be adapted to the force of the fever and re-active power of the patient. A feeble child, or patient of any age, must not be permanently chilled. Less water and more warm-handed friction.

Scrofula is said to be derived from *scrofa,* a sow, because it is a disease of swine, and one occasioned by feeding like hogs, or upon hogs. It is a hereditary disease, or may be developed by diseasing causes. It causes arrest of development, accumulations of morbid matter, inflammation, softening, and destruction of all the tissues of the body. Scrofulous infants have small

limbs, large abdomens, protruding chests, large heads
weak spines, and are liable to ulcerations and hernia
Its ravages begin before birth, and end only with death.
Lugol estimates that one quarter of all scrofulous children are destroyed by spontaneous abortion. Scrofulous infants die of convulsions, and dropsy of the brain,
cholera infantum, consumption of the lungs, bowels,
and spine, and scrofula makes all diseases dangerous.
In the mucous membranes it causes sore eyes, running
from the nose and ears, worms, whites, diarrhœa, etc.
In the skin it produces chilblains, eruptions of the eyelids and around the ears; pustules on the face and
chest; tubercles and abscesses in the cellular tissue;
rickets and rotting of the bones; tubercular consumption of the lungs, liver, and every soft organ of the
body. In fact, according to Lugol, the accumulation
of morbid matter, in the form of tubercle, is the great
characteristic of this disease.

We cannot always tell what determines the disease
to any particular organ. Of several scrofulous children,
one may have ophthalmia, one rickets, a third enlargement of the glands of the neck, or king's evil; others
cutaneous affections, deep ulcers, white swelling, hip-
disease, convulsions, hydrocephalus, pulmonary consumption, etc., etc., but it is all one disease—all scrofula.
This disease accompanies, and is, doubtless, caused by,
activity and excess in the generative function. The
too great amativeness of parents produces scrofulous
children, who, inheriting the disease of the passion, as
well as the organism, develop the latter by the former.
So goes on this work of death.

Scrofula destroys its victims every stage. There are
abortions in gestation; deaths from all the diseases of
infancy, and in youth the various forms of consumption.
Whatever part is weakest, or becomes in any way diseased, becomes the focus of scrofula. If such a child
takes cold, it dies of chronic bronchitis, or pneumonia;

some irritation or over-action causes determination to the brain, and we have brain fever, tubercles, convulsions, effusion, and death; the bowels are disordered, and there sets in an incurable diarrhœa or dysentery, or some trifling injury develops disease of the elbow joint, white swelling of the knee, or hip disease.

Causes.—Lugol believes scrofula to be always hereditary. I believe the disease may be developed first, and then transmitted. Children are born scrofulous when their parents have had syphilis, or have been licentious; are too young or too old, or of disproportionate ages or strength; are nearly related; or suffer from any of the causes of disease. Scrofula, I believe, also arises in men, as in animals, from darkness, bad air, bad food, such as the milk of scrofulous nurses and badly kept and fed cows; from eating pork and the flesh of other diseased animals.

To prevent scrofula, we must abolish all its causes, abolish poverty, abolish filth, abolish vice, abolish drugs, abolish all that poisons, weakens, and degrades humanity. We must teach mankind the laws, and surround them with the conditions, of health.

Treatment.—Light, air, exercise, cleanliness, a pure moderate diet, and all healthy conditions, with an avoidance of all causes of disease, especially in the exercise, natural or otherwise, of the generative system, with the water-cure and all its powerful means of invigoration and purification.

Take a full morning bath, with much friction; mid forenoon, a dripping sheet; mid afternoon, a wet-sheet pack one day, and the next a dry blanket pack, or the wet-sheet pack two days, and blanket pack on the third day; all packs long and thorough; at night wear a bandage from the hips to the armpits.

Such a course as this, or as thorough an one as the strength of the patient can bear, will wash the disease

R

out of the system, if it has not already produced fatal disorganisation.

When there is local scrofulous disease, the treatment must still be general. Cold applications to the part excite the diseased action. We must pay especial attention to secure a healthy nutrition. The food cannot be too pure and simple. It should consist of fruit and farinacea, with soft water to drink. Grapes, strawberries, and similar sub-acid fruits are excellent. Plenty of grapes will alone go far to effect a cure.

The scrofulous matter, with this treatment, *does come out*. It exudes from every pore. Sometimes it comes out in eruptions, or boils, filled with the characteristic matter; and whether the matter comes out by the pores, or a pint at a time from abscesses, the result is purifi cation, and purification is health.

All general poisonings of the system, as by opium, tobacco, coffee, tea, ardent spirits, mercury, lead, quinine, syphilis, are to be treated upon the same principles as scrofula.

Scurvy, hydrophobia, glanders, cancer, rheumatism, and the more external affections, as salt rheum, psora, impetigo, and the whole list of skin diseases, are subject to the same laws, and require, with simple and obvious modifications, the same course of invigoration and purification. I shall speak of many of these separately, but I group them here to illustrate a principle.

CHAPTER XVIII.

INFLAMMATION AND BRAIN DISEASES.

Inflammation.—As inflammation is the essential constituent of nearly all acute diseases, and lays the
foundation of nearly all chronic affections, an understanding of its nature, causes, effects, and treatment,
will make the rest of my task an easy one.

Inflammation is characterised by four signs—heat,
redness, pain, and swelling.   But either may exist
alone without inflammation.   There may be redness
from blushing, heat, or friction; pain may be neuralgic,
or spasmodic, in which cases it is diminished by
pressure; swelling may be dropsical.

The exciting causes of inflammation are heat, cold,
injuries; the real or pre-disposing cause lies deeper.
In a pure and vigorous system, neither heat, nor cold,
nor injuries cause inflammations.   The most terrible
wounds heal rapidly, and with no bad effects; while
in an impure and debilitated system, a slight chill will
produce an inflammation of the lungs, and a slight
injury the swelling of an entire limb.   We have, then,
the same causes for inflammation as for fever; and
fever, as I said before, is only a general inflammation,
and inflammation is only a circumscribed fever.

Inflammation may terminate spontaneously, by the
return of the part affected to its natural state; this is
resolution, by an increase of the natural discharges,
as in catarrh, diarrhœa, dysentery, gleet, etc., and by
dropsy; by schirrus, or an indolent hardening, with
shooting pain, liable to become cancerous; by hemorrhage in vascular parts; by metastasis, or the shifting of
the disease from one region to another; by suppuration,
or the formation of pus; by gangrene, or mortification.

Inflammation of a part may also be attended or followed by the formation of various tumours, or morbid growths, mild or malignant; and by the gathering of scrofulous, or other matter of disease.

In all cases, inflammation is the act of the part affected. The blood is summoned to it, and retained in it. The nervous power increases capillary action, by which heat is evolved, and the pressure upon, or distention of, the nerves of sensation, causes the pain. All this is for something. The increased flow of blood to a part brings an increase of morbid matter, and that calls for an increased effort to dislodge it. Calomel is washed through the parotid glands in floods of saliva; foul matter runs from the nose and air passages in an increased flow of mucus; it is poured through the intestinal glands in a diarrhœa; from the kidneys in diabetes; or, when deeper seated, and harder to dislodge, it comes out in purulent secretions. A foreign body in the flesh is removed, brought to the surface, and cast out by this process. Not long ago, a lady near Manchester, in a fit of mania, swallowed a dessert knife seven inches long. Inflammation was set up, and it was safely cast out of the abdomen near the umbilicus.

A full diet promotes inflammation, because the organic powers, which should be engaged in freeing the system of its impure matter, are expended in digesting and conveying away unnecessary food. It is in this way that every ounce more than a man requires is an injury. It takes vital force that is needed for other uses. A clean, abstemious man—in a word, a healthy man—is not liable to inflammations. The law of inflammation is the same as fever, and its treatment is to be governed by the same principles.

If an inflammation is external, we may generally cut it short at the beginning by the application of extreme cold, as ice, or ice-water. If internal, our

method is to derive to the surface, and relieve the
inflamed part, by drawing the blood away, and
opening other avenues for the excretion of morbid
matter. By this means, we produce an artificial
metastasis, as when we relieve an internal inflammation by bringing out an eruption on the skin. This
is the use of blisters. The objection to them is
needless violence, and the poisonous means by which
they are produced. A mustard poultice, the mustard
paper, or mustard sprinkled on compress, or pack,
hastens the relief of internal inflammation. Sharp
friction with a flesh brush answers a similar purpose.

Sometimes inflammation is reduced by applying
cold to the part affected, and warmth to some other
near or distant part. An ingenious remedy for felon,
in its early stage, is to place the elbow in very warm
water, and apply, at the same time, ice-water to the
finger. Inflammation of the brain is also met by
putting the feet and legs in hot water, and applying
cold-water to the head.

The wet-sheet pack, as an equaliser of the circulation, is the best of all remedies for inflammation of
any part, external or internal—from a finger or toe, to
the lungs or brain. The half-bath may be, in some
cases, a more rapid and powerful remedy ; but it is not
of such universal application.

The first stage of inflammation is called congestion.
It is the gathering of the blood in the part, before the
diseased action is fully established. In this stage,
relief is easily effected, but when there is induration it
cannot be overcome so quickly, and suppuration must
take its natural course.

Inflammation of the Brain or its membranes, is
characterised by great heat, fulness, violent pain,
suffusion of the face, redness of the eyes, vomiting,
general fever, delirium ; then stupor, fixedness of the

pupils, coma ; rigidity or convulsion of the muscles ; followed by relaxation and death.

The treatment is the application of cold to the head in the most decided and thorough manner, with warmth and friction to the lower part of the body. I have kept the head encased in snow for six hours, with the body in a wet-sheet pack.

Pathologists distinguish between congestion and inflammation of the brain and its membranes, each membrane, and even the different portions of each ; but there is no practical benefit in these niceties. If there is acute inflammation within the cranium, we have but one means of meeting it.

Chronic Inflammation of the Brain is characterised by the various symptoms of insanity. Water has been used for ages for the treatment of this disease, and sometimes with good effect. I have great faith in its continued persevering application, and hope to see it fairly tried in some of our insane asylums. A daily bath, pack, and injections, with all healthy conditions, and a pure vegetable diet, would give promise of cure.

Insanity appears often to be a disease of exhaustion, as it is caused by masturbation. It is also excited by disappointed love, grief, and various discordances of the passions. The risk of it is greatly increased by hereditary predisposition.

Delirium Tremens is a form of insanity, depending upon an exhausted and irritable condition of the brain. It is caused by the use of intoxicating drinks. Milder forms of nervous irritation come from the use of tobacco, tea, coffee, and opium.

A half-bath, or a wet-sheet pack, is a sovereign soother of nervous irritability. In severe cases of mania, or delirium tremens, the half-bath should be used perseveringly, with frequent cold affusions to the head.

Apoplexy is a sudden paralysis, insensibility, or stupor, resembling deep sleep, with full breathing, and regular pulse, commonly resulting in palsy or death. It is caused by pressure on the brain, either distention of the blood-vessels, effusion of serum, or effusion of blood. It is a disease of exhaustion, and generally of old age. Men who have worked with their brains, using stimulants, and eating too much, are most subject to this disease.

The only reasonable treatment is the application of cold to the head, and warmth to the extremities. This may relieve and cure, if there is no actual effusion.

When the patient survives the first attack, and is left with paralysis of one side of the body, a thorough course of invigorating treatment, with a strict diet, and absolute temperance and continence, may restore him to health.

Apoplexy so much resembles drunkenness, that it cannot always be distinguished; it is also closely simulated by paroxysms of hysteria.

Paralysis is a disease, either of the brain, the spinal cord, or of the nerves. It is a loss of action, from oppression or exhaustion.

Hemiplegia is paralysis of one half the body, caused by pressure or atony of the opposite side of the brain.

Paraplegia is palsy of the lower part of the body, from some point in the spinal column.

Shaking Palsy is a general partial paralysis in exhaustion, generally from old age.

Paralysis may affect a single organ, limb, or muscle; it may also affect either the nerves of motion or sensation, or both. It is generally, however, in the nerves of motion. It is seldom complete; and in hemiplegia, we find the arm worse than the leg, simply because the latter has been more exercised.

The two causes of palsy are exhaustion and poisoning. The exhaustion generally comes from amative indulgence, the poisoning from tobacco, but the exhaustion *may* come from any labour or excitement of body or mind, and the poisoning from food, drink, bad air, etc. The two great causes, however, of all this class of diseases, are licentiousness and tobacco. It is seldom that we see women affected with them, because they seldom indulge in both, if they do in either.

Paraplegia may come from disease or injury of the spine, or from some derangement of the digestive organs; more commonly from the latter.

These diseases are seldom cured : but here, as everywhere, the water and hygienic treatment have had their triumphs. We must govern our applications by the age and vitality of the patient, and also by the causes of disease. If there is exhaustion, we must give invigorating treatment—if poisoning, we must wash the offending matter from the system. In every case there must be a careful diet, and the best possible conditions. The wet-sheet pack, the douche, long continued friction with the hands of strong persons, are the best remedies. The palsied limbs must be regularly exercised. Galvanic currents are powerful stimulants of nervous action ; but I cannot see that such currents are produced by what are called galvanic chains or bands. Animal magnetism, or the direct transfer of nervous force from a strong person to a weak one is one of the best of remedies.

Chorea Sancta Vita, or St. Vitus's Dance, is a disease of childhood or youth, and is produced in nine cases in ten, by solitary amative indulgence. Sometimes it is attributed to worms, or other irritations of the digestive organs. It yields readily to a strict diet, wet-sheet pack, sitz-baths, the douche upon the spine, and injections, if the cause is removed.

Epilepsy is one of the most terrible of this class of diseases. The patient is suddenly, with or without warning, attacked by violent convulsions, foaming at the mouth, grinding the teeth, with every appearance of agony, but no after memory of suffering. The fit lasts from ten minutes to an hour. Sometimes there are several in succession. These paroxysms may occur daily, several times a-day, or at intervals of weeks or months.

Epileptic fits are caused in infants by dentition or worms; they sometimes precede or follow eruptive fevers; but there are few of epilepsy that are not caused by amative excess or masturbation. In some cases, tobacco, ardent spirits, and dietetic irregularities have lent their aid.

The treatment is the absolute avoidance of these causes of disease, a strict diet, and full treatment, especially that of an invigorating character. Coarse bread, or wheat meal porridge, and fruit, with sitz-baths and injections, should secure the action of the bowels. I cannot too strongly urge the necessity of continence and the most careful diet. When the patient has been going on well for some time, a single amative indulgence, social or solitary, or the least variation from a strict diet, in quantity or quality, may cause a fit. Sometimes a fit may be prevented by a strong mesmerising.

Catalepsy, or trance, is a spasm or paralysis of the nerves of motion and general sensation all over the body. Consciousness is often retained, and the cataleptic may know everything that is going on, while his friends believe him to be dead. So complete, in some cases, is the suspension of all apparent vitality, that many persons have been buried alive in this state. Sometimes the soul seems to have a supernatural activity, and visions of the spiritual world are related by those who have been in this condition.

The treatment can only be directed to the general health of the patient.

Neuralgia.—Under this name may be included those

painful affections which are not connected with any apparent organic lesion. Spinal irritation is an obscure pain and weakness in the back, extending down the thighs. Tic Doloureux is pain in the expansion of some external nerve, usually of the face. Visceral neuralgia is a paroxysmal and recurrent affection of the nerves of internal organs. Sciatica is neural in the back of the hip and thigh.

What are the causes of neuralgia? Every cause of general disease may produce this particular development. Its centre is dyspepsia. It is caused by nervous exhaustion of any kind, or from any cause. Tea, coffee, tobacco, high living, bad air, all unhealthy habits, and particularly all exhausting passions, produce this disease. It has been cured by surgical operations, pulling teeth, or cutting off nerves; but the last often fails from the nerve re-uniting. Abstinence from all causes of disease is a cure. Cold water, even in a local application, has cured cases which defied all the usual remedies. The wet-sheet pack relieves and cures. In severe cases we must use all means of purification and invigoration. If it comes from dyspepsia, we must cure that; if from uterine or ovarian disease, that must be attended to. The local affection, when it can be reached, may always be relieved by intense cold.

Gout and Rheumatism are nearly allied to these nervous diseases. Gout is hereditary, and so, to some extent, is its milder neighbour. Gout is mostly confined to the joints, especially of the extremities, and usually attacks those of the great toe. Rheumatism attacks every part of the body. Each is believed to leave external for internal organs, so that we hear of gout in the stomach and rheumatism in the heart. Both change rapidly from one part to another. Gouty patients are liable to violent affections of the brain, heart, lungs, stomach, etc.

When Harvey had the gout, he resolutely plunged

the affected foot into a pail of the coldest water he could find. I believe that there was no more danger than in any other species of inflammation. Strict temperance, passional and dietetic, with exercise, is generally a preventive. In some cases, hereditary predispositions are very strong, but as a rule, no one suffers from gout without indolence or excess. The gouty patient must bring himself into healthy conditions, and he will generally banish the gout. It may be relieved by the cold bath to the part, the wet bandage, and the wet-sheet pack. A gouty patient needs a full course of water-cure treatment; but he will get well if he follows an old prescription—"Live on sixpence a-day, and earn it."

Acute Rheumatism comes on with stiffness and pain in the joints or muscles, followed by fever. The pain is severe, the part swollen and red; the pulse full, hard, and frequent, the tongue lightly furred, the skin harsh, hot, and dry. It lasts ten or twelve days, and then slowly subsides. It is a disease of excess in diet, stimulants, and amative indulgence, with bad air, and want of proper exercise. It commonly occurs in young persons of full habit.

Treatment the same as for fever, with wet bandages to the parts affected. In these cases, the cold, full, double, and treble wet-sheet pack is "heaven" to the patient. It is better than all the opium in the world. With a course of thorough and frequent packing, the system is thoroughly purified. Its prevention is as evident and easy as that of the gout.

Chronic Rheumatism is a disease "better felt than expressed," and too common to render any description necessary. It is the disease of exhaustion and age. It produces shrinking of the muscles, and swelling and stiffness of the joints. Some poor patients are drawn into terrible distortions. Lumbago is rheumatism of the small of the back.

A careful, moderate diet, alternate packing with the wet-sheet and blanket pack, inducing thorough sweating with the latter, drinking water, and plenty of rubbing, will cure any case of rheumatism, when the patient has strength enough left to be cured. When the joints are stiffening, they must be moved, even if the pain is severe. Stimulating bandages may be worn almost continually upon the parts affected. Counter irritation with sharp flesh-brush or mustard often relieves. The Turkish and vapour baths are also well suited to this class of disorders.

CHAPTER XIX.

DISEASES OF THE ORGANS OF RESPIRATION.

THIS class of diseases destroys nearly half of all civilised races, so vital a thing is it to breathe. In the earliest infancy, death is sometimes caused by inflammation of the lungs, from the mere contact of the air with its delicate, half-formed tissues. Tubercular consumption also occurs in infancy. Then comes that terror of mothers, croup. Hooping-cough is sometimes fatal. Further along comes bronchitis, pneumonia, pleurisy, the tubercular phthisis of early middle age, and asthma.

The lungs are made up of air-vessels, blood-vessels, and nerves. Their healthy condition requires good air and a free respiration, pure blood, and a free circulation, and sufficient nervous energy. Disease comes from the lack of either, or all of these conditions.

Croup is an inflammation of the larynx, extending to the trachea. It usually attacks children of one year old and upward. Its signs are, difficult breathing, with cough and fever. It usually comes on toward evening, with the appearance of a common cold, sneezing, etc. The breathing becomes rapidly more difficult, the face is red, the eyes suffused; the patient sits up in bed, and struggles for breath. The cough, and finally the breathing, has a peculiar sound, called "croupy." A false membrane is formed in the throat, and that, with the swelling of the larynx, chokes the patient to death.

This is a disease of scrofulous, fat, over-fed, and delicately reared children. No child, with a moderately good constitution, who takes exercise outdoors, breathes good air night and day, eats moderately of simple healthy food, and is washed all over every morning in cold water, ever dies of croup. In some cases of delicate children, the disease comes on so insidiously, that the membrane is formed almost before its nature is suspected.

No disease is more simple to treat, or, taken in season, easier to cure. It is a simple inflammation of an organ within our reach; and the treatment is the immediate, continued, and thorough application of the coldest water to the throat. Apply this for fifteen minutes, with friction over the throat and chest, and follow by a partial or full wet-sheet pack, according to the fever. Renew the cold by a compress to the throat, in the pack. Repeat the whole, if necessary, but it seldom will be. The pack, as in all cases, to be followed by a wash-down, and in this case, much friction. A strict diet, morning bath, and cold affusion and rubbing of the throat for a week, completes the cure. The thorough washing of the throat with cold water is a prevention against this and all throat diseases.

Diphtheria is similar to croup, in that a false membrane is formed in the throat; but it is a disease of a lower, more chronic, but not less fatal type. The treatment cannot, therefore be so heroic. The wet-sheet pack, with full perspirations at an early stage gives the best chance of cure. But it is in regard to these insidious and generally fatal diseases that prevention is all important. A really healthy child does not have croup or diphtheria.

Acute Bronchitis is an inflammation of the mucous membrane, lining the air passages of the lungs. We may include the trachea, as the beginning of these tubes. It begins like any common cold; there is sore throat, and a dry, tickling cough; fever follows, with a harsh, hot skin, flushed face, pain in the back and limbs, difficult breathing, tightness across the chest, pain in coughing, crepitous rattle through the thorax. As the expectoration becomes free, these symptoms subsid . Scrofulous or any other impurity of constitution predisposes to this disease.

The treatment is the wet-sheet pack, and blanket pack alternately; with the wet bandage, or jacket around the lungs at night, well covered; with all other ,ealthy conditions, and *absolute diet*, which means cold water *ad libitum*, and nothing else. Resolution is much promoted by friction of the chest, with a coarse towel, hair mitten, or flesh brush.

Chronic Bronchitis.—This disease is merely a mild and continued form of the above, going on gradually to the thickening of the membrane, interference with the objects of respiration, consequent emaciation, quick pulse, fever, night-sweats, and other hectic symptoms At a certain stage it is as hopeless as phthisis.

In all these affections of the throat and lungs the expectoration may be mucous, muco-purulent, or purulent. Pus is no special sign of tubercular disease. It may occur on any inflamed surface, as well as in deep ulcers or abscess. When large quantities of pus are thrown off suddenly, we know it comes from abscess

Bakers, stone-cutters, and others engaged in dusty and unhealthy employments are subject to this disease.

Treatment the same as in the acute form, modified

to suit the strength and re-active power of the patient. The wet jacket may be worn all the time with great advantage. Any action of the skin relieves, if relief is possible. But some cases resist all our efforts. Where there is extensive thickening of the mucous membrane, or hardening of the substance of the lung, the result must be fatal.

Pleurisy and Pneumonia—the inflammation of the lining membrane of the lungs, and of their substance—are so connected in their nature, causes, and treatment, that we need not consider them apart. In the first the pain is acute, hindering the action of the chest; in the latter it is deeper and duller, accompanied by a difficult respiration.

In inflammation of the lungs, we have several stages; congestion, marked by oppression; inflammation, with dull pain and reddish expectoration; hepatisation, or hardening, with little expectoration; softening, with increased and reddish expectoration; resolutions, with mucous expectoration. There is much fever and great distress.

Acute pneumonia may terminate in sudden death by loss of function, in abscess, or in the chronic form of the disease, when it is often mistaken for phthisis.

Pleurisy may end in effusion of water in the chest, in effusion of pus, and the formation of adhesions; all dangerous. The general causes of these diseases are not different from those of all the affections of these organs. Their exciting cause is commonly cold, especially following exhaustion.

The treatment is absolute diet, cold sponging of the chest, the wet compress, and the wet-sheet pack. Alternate and repeat these incessantly. Pleurisy may be cut short by a vigorous application of cold to the affected region, as in croup; but when pneumonia has advanced beyond its first stage, it requires at least six days for its resolution.

These, and most internal conjestions and inflammations may often be speedily relieved by counter-irritation, with mustard, or by the application of cloths dipped in hot water and put on for a few minutes as hot as they can be borne. After the first relief the packs and free perspirations complete the cure.

Spitting of Blood.—Hemorrhage is unpleasant under all circumstances, and is often a sign of danger; but, in most cases, it is not of so much importance as the patient imagines. Nose-bleed is frequent in delicate and plethoric constitutions, and is brought on by any excitement. Thoroughly bathing the head and neck, and snuffing cold water up the nostrils, generally cures it.

The saliva is often tinged with blood from the gums, or a decayed tooth. This may be distinguished from bleeding from the lungs, or air passages, by there being no cough. When blood comes with coughing, its source is below the glottis, or opening into the larynx. When it comes from the upper part of the pharynx, or around the fauces, it is merely hawked up Blood from the stomach can come up in no way but by eructation or vomiting, and it is usually dark coloured.

Blood may come from the whole extent of the organs of respiration, in several ways. In weakness, and congestion of the mucous membrane, of any part, there may be simple exudation from the small vessels. There may be bleeding high in the throat, from speaking, coughing, or blowing on some musical instrument. This is of no consequence, but as a sign of weakness, and liability to more serious disease. In many persons there is a constitutional weakness in the blood-vessels which makes them liable to hemorrhages. They spit blood all their lives.

Pulmonary apoplexy is a sudden congestion of some portion of the lungs, with a feeling of fulness and suffocation. The blood-vessels are engorged, and crowd upon the air-vessels, so that they cannot be filled. This state may be caused by any excitement, but is especially the result of grief, or other depressing passions. Sometimes it passes off gradually, without loss of blood; often it is relieved by a more or less extensive hemorrhage. The blood gushes into the air-passages, and is coughed up.

In abscess of the lungs, from inflammation or tubercle, hemorrhage arises from some blood-vessel being involved in the abscess. Nature does much in these cases to protect herself; but she sometimes wants the strength to do it effectually. She always makes the effort, first to form the abscess as far as possible from large vessels, and secondly, to thicken or close up those that are involved. But sometimes a severe fit of coughing breaks them apart, and there is more or less bleeding.

The treatment in all these cases must be soothing, cooling, and derivative. A wet compress may be laid upon the throat and chest, while the lower extremities are well rubbed, or put in hot water.

In all cases of tendency to pulmonary apoplexy, or bleeding from the lungs from any cause, severe chills must be avoided. A too cold sitz-bath, a cold half-bath, or staying too long in the plunge bath, have caused congestion of the lungs and hemorrhage. Heroism is a fine thing—heroic treatment in water-cure is sometimes the best thing—but it is not safe in all cases. For heroic treatment we must have heroic constitutions, and these are not so plentiful as could be wished.

Asthma is a distressing, paroxysmal, periodic, or recurrent disease, the chief feature of which is great difficulty of breathing. Its nature is not well understood. It is supposed to be spasmodic; entirely functional in the beginning, but finally causing organic

S

changes. I believe it to be originally an affection of the pneumo-gastric nerves. It is clearly hereditary.

There are curious differences in the exciting causes. In some, the fits are brought on by the smoky, thick air of a city; others have them when they go to the country. Many cannot sleep in the neighbourhood of certain trees, as the alanthus. But there is one feature which I believe is never absent. The asthmatic patient is always dyspeptic, and any degree of gastric irritation promotes the recurrence of the paroxysms. A single meal of hot bread or pastry, or other indigestible food, will bring forty-eight hours of agony.

Cure the dyspepsia and you cure the asthma. Taking proper care in other respects, you have two great points to effect—two great organs to relieve—the stomach and the skin. I have never seen a case of asthma which could not be relieved; and the worst cases were cured by packing and a strict diet. Whoever will resolutely starve and bathe, or, still better, take packs, may be cured. But it is of little use to try the water, if the diet is not attended to. In one case, I was able to give only blanket packs, followed by a full cold bath, and much rubbing. Every sweat acted like a charm.

Consumption is a name which applies to any wasting disease, but it is specially confined to diseases of the lungs. Considering chronic bronchitis as a separate disease, we may restrict the designation to pulmonary abscess, from pneumonia or tubercle. The latter is called phthisis, or scrofulous consumption; though scrofula may be as clearly the cause of abscess from inflammation as tubercle. In every case, there is a destruction of the lungs from the gathering of morbid matter.

Consumption is a disease of hereditary taint and pre-disposition. The very germ or zoosperm, is tainted, diseased, scrofulous, and consumptive. Nature, in all cases, makes an effort to protect her new beings, and this effort is often successful. The child may be saved from its parents' diseases. The placenta may protect the foetus from the morbid matters in the blood of the mother. The scrofulous matter may be expelled by the diseases of infancy. These things take place under favourable circumstances.

Abscess from inflammation of the lungs is not necessarily fatal. It may break into the pleural cavity, and the pus be absorbed, or find an outward opening, or it may open into the air passages, and be thrown off by expectoration, the cavity gradually contracting and cicatrising, as in any other organ. On the other hand, where the system is weak and full of impurities, the abscess may be kept open, and the strength fail from continued irritation and exhausting action. In this case there will be hectic, emaciation, diarrhœa, dropsy, and death.

Tubercular consumption begins by the deposition of minute, or, as they are called, milliary tubercles in the lungs, usually in the upper portion, just under the collar bone. These are sometimes found in a new born infant. They spread, increase in size, soften, suppurate, form ulcers, and their matter is thrown off. Sometimes many join together to form a large ulcer.

The first effect of tubercle is to render a portion of the lungs useless for the purposes of respiration. This quickens the pulse and shortens the breath, and there is consequent weakness and feverishness. The little, dry, hacking cough, which marks the first stages of this disease, seems to come from the irritation of foreign matter, the invasion of a portion of the lungs, and an instinctive effort to expel it. Every stage of the progress of consumption is an effort to cure, and this effort is sometimes effectual. In many cases where consumption has not been suspected, there are found in the lungs after death, unmistakeable signs of former tubercles, which have softened, been expelled, and healed. But in the majority of cases, there is too much disease, and too little vital force.

The signs of tubercular consumption are a delicate, scrofulous appearance; narrow chest; dry, hacking cough; pain in the chest; languor; debility; emaciation; quick pulse; hurried respiration; dry, hot hand, or cold hands and feet; panting and palpitation on running up stairs; purulent expectoration; hectic fever; diarrhœa; swelling of the ankles; atrophy; marasmus.

Cheerfulness and hope of recovery are remarkable symptoms, and generally present unless there is dyspepsia.

There are cases of consumption going on to a fatal termination, in which most of the characteristic symptoms are wanting.

The causes of consumption have been already referred to. It is to a remarkable extent hereditary. All the causes of scrofula are causes of consumption. None are so liable to it as those who have wasted their lives in masturbation or sexual excess. The two causes of this, as of all diseases, are exhaustion and impurity. The causes which especially affect the lungs, such as tight lacing, bad air, irritating substances, are all causes of consumption. Its access is hastened by frequent colds, exposure to a damp, cold atmosphere, cold feet, and all causes which tend to irritate, inflame, or congest the respiratory system.

Whole families die of consumption; it is developed in many persons who are subjected to the same causes, or who live in the same habits; it is possible that constant proximity may produce similar constitutional conditions and tendencies. It is probable that it can be communicated by innoculation, and by inhaling the dried expectorations of consumptive patients. Syphilis causes scrofula—scrofula produces tubercle.

Can consumption be cured? Hundreds of quacks, regular and irregular, draw revenues from millions of victims, by flattering the hopes which belong to this disease, with an affirmative answer. I, too, must say, *consumption can be cured; has been cured; will be cured.* It is curable in its early stages ; curable when but a small portion of the lungs is involved; curable where there is a moderate amount of disease, and much vigour to combat it. But where it has gone on to a certain point of weakness; where a large portion of the lungs is tuberculated ; where there is much disease and little vitality, it is of necessity fatal. Nature cannot effect a cure, and art has no miraculous power. In this, as in all cases, we must depend upon the vital forces.

The cure cannot be too soon commenced. We must begin with birth. No infant should be allowed to suck a scrofulous mother or nurse. If a perfectly healthy, cleanly, proper nurse cannot be procured—one that has a good constitution, and will observe all the laws of health—a good cow, which lives in good air and on good food, is much better.

A pure diet, a pure air at all times, daily bathing in cold water, and much exercise in the open air, are all absolute necessities. If any sign of scrofula is developed, go through a course of thorough wet-sheet packing, and bring it to the surface. Every night put a wet bandage around the abdomen. See that the spine is straight and the lungs expanded. Banish tight dressing, corsets, and all fashionable abominations. See that the child sleeps on a cool, hard bed, without too much covering. Especially see that this child of your heart fall into no destructive habit. Don't presume that he or she will not—make sure of it. A child of a year old may get into this habit, either from some perverted instinct or from some irritation of the genital organs. This is especially the case with little girls. There is an itching ; the friction used to allay it produces a certain result—it is repeated, and the habit is formed, the nervous system wrecked. Many sweet and innocent children fall into this most exhausting vice. Every child, male or female, should be carefully watched, until it is old enough to understand the subject, and then it should be carefully explained to it. The earlier this is done, and the stronger the impression made upon the mind of the child of the wickedness of this abuse, the better. It is truly a matter of life and death; and squeamishness is as much out of place as if the child were dying.

When the disease has begun, and in any of its stages, the patient must be placed in all healthy conditions, especially those of pure air, light, exercise, and cleanliness. I have no doubt that a purely vegetable diet, or one of bread, milk, and fruits, is the best. Even the milk may not be so well as pure, soft water; it certainly is not, if its quality is doubtful; above all, the quantity must be small. We must invigorate by daily full baths; we must purify by as much packing as the patient can bear. The wet-jacket may be worn night and day. Sweating is of advantage, if the patient can bear it. The dripping sheet or cold sponging is good for the night-sweats; cold water injections for the diarrhœa.

By these means many have been saved. Some have been cured, who seemed marked for death; others have had their lives prolonged, and made comfortable for months and years.

No drug ever cured consumption—most drugs in allopathic doses are mischievous, and none is more so than that which is almost universally given, and which enters largely into the composition of nearly all the nostrums in use. I mean opium. After a time all the soothing effects of opium are lost, and the disease is made more painful.

Change of climate may be favourable. A soft, dry,

pure air is better than a harsh, damp, impure one.   But I distrust the enervating effects of warm climates.   In a mild one, the patient gains by being much in the open air.   Change of scene may remove some cause of disease, but going north may be as well as going south. Some think a cold air better than a warm one.   It may be, if you can be out of doors.   There seems no doubt that a dry atmosphere is better than one loaded with damps and fogs.   When we have lost the use of any portion of the lungs, we should get the best air we can, and breathe as much of it as possible.   High and dry, pure and warm places seem best for most consumptives.   Horseback exercise is among the most favourable.   I think much of strengthening the chest by exercises, and systematic, deep breathing.

Eat pure food, and not too much.   Use up no vital force in digesting and excreting unnecessary food. Breathe pure air, much of it; the blood wants all the oxygen it can get.   Keep the skin clean, and promote its activity.   Live out of doors, in the light and air ; and give Nature a fair chance to save her child.   Rely upon her, as a mother, who will do all that can be done for her offspring.   Do the best you can, make a good fight for life, and then bravely and patiently accept your fate.

CHAPTER XX.

DISEASES OF THE ORGANS OF DIGESTION.

As the beautiful development and healthy vigour of the whole system, animal and organic, depends upon the proper performance of the function of nutrition, especially in its earlier processes of digestion and assimilation, it is evident that any disease of the digestive organs, or any disturbance of their function, must be of the first importance. There are many such diseases, or forms and localities of disease; but I shall begin with one that is central and pervading — the monster disease of civilisation, and the cause or complication of almost every other.

Dyspepsia is more than a disease of the stomach, and means more than indigestion. It is a disease of both sexes, all ages, and all conditions. Infants are born with it—aged people die of it.

Its symptoms are legion, if we give this name to all its effects. Among them are a morbid appetite, acid eructations, heart-burn, a painful fulness, distention or weight of the stomach, nausea, vomiting, emaciation, flatulence, colics, constipation, diarrhœa, general debility, languor, great depression of spirits, vertigo, headache, dim and depraved vision, sleeplessness, nocturnal restlessness, hypo, palpitation of the heart, slow or intermittent pulse, foul, white, furred, or red and deeply-furrowed tongue, bad teeth, fœtid breath, pimples, a greasy, dull complexion, pallor, sallowness, dulness of all the senses, loss of all faculties, insanity, suicide, etc., etc. This list might be prolonged to an indefinite extent.

The seat of the disease is the central ganglia of the organic system of nerves, which preside over the secretion of the gastric juice, and generally over the digestive and assimilative processes. Every other organ of the body is affected either by nervous relation and sympathy, or by the morbid condition of the blood. The causes, effects, and relations of dyspepsia cover almost the whole ground of pathology. Abernethy, when called to an ulcer, or a sore toe, always went to work at the stomach as the centre of disease, though not always in the most judicious way, according to my "humble opinion."

Dyspepsia may be hereditary. It may come from either parent. We have no occasion to doubt this; for children "take after" their parents in much less important particulars

The diet of the nurse may give an infant dyspepsia. Whatever will give the mother or nurse this disease, will so affect the milk as to cause it in the child.

Eating too much food will cause dyspepsia, by overtasking the power of the stomach to digest and dispose of surplus food, and by the undigested food lying in the stomach, a source of irritation. Eating too fast, by preventing mastication and insalivation. Those who eat too fast, generally eat too much. Eating hot food and drinking hot drinks, which enfeeble the stomach. Eating indigestible food, as new bread, short-cakes, pastry, sweetmeats, pickles, oily and greasy meats, gravies, mince-pies, and *all that sort of thing*. We exhaust the power of an organ, if we overtask it—we disease it, if we task it unnaturally. Eating condiments, as pepper, ginger, mustard, spices. Taking drugs. Every poison taken into the stomach must injure it. All spirituous and narcotic-beverages, tea, coffee, and alcoholic drinks. Tobacco, above all, by its direct action upon the nervous system, by its acrid, irritating character, and by its constant excitement of the salivary glands and waste of this secretion. Even a constant loss of saliva, as by spinners in moistening linen, will produce dyspepsia; much more the spitting of the smoker and chewer.

Any kind of exhaustion, by bodily labour, action, or anxiety of mind; sedentary occupation; absorption in business; circumstances of depression, all cause dyspepsia. It is especially a disease of exhaustion.

Let a man eat a hearty meal, and then take violent exercise, or go to work, or get excited, or hear bad news, and digestion is suspended. Frequent repetition of this will cause dyspepsia.

When the process of digestion begins, the vital power gathers around the digestive organs. The blood goes to the stomach. The force of the system is centred there. Now, if this be drawn off, or divided, the work is badly done, if done at all; the blood is poor and half vitalised; poor blood makes poor gastric juice; poor gastric juice makes poor blood; and so it goes on in a progression of badness. Now, add to all these causes one more—exhaustion from amativeness, solitary or social, and you are near the root of evil.

Exhaustion calls for too much food, and stimulating food. Too much food produces exhaustion.

Let us see how dyspeptics are made. A man, in New York, gets up late in the morning, exhausted by a night's excess, takes no bath, hurries down to breakfast, bolts hot rolls or buckwheat cakes saturated with butter, ham and eggs, sausages, and a few other abominations, washes them down with two cups of hot coffee, lights his cigar, and hurries down town; goes to work fiercely, with an occasional cigar, till twelve or one o'clock; rushes out, and into some eating-house; bolts a rapid meal of meat, gravy, condiments, pastry, ale, or brandy; more cigars; back to work like a steam-engine; home in the omnibus, to a luxurious dinner; theatre; oyster supper; brandy and cigars; bed at midnight, with a feverish excitement made up of beef, brandy, oysters, coffee, and tobacco, prompting to amative indulgence and more exhaustion. Try this two or three years, and see if all the resources of nature will save you from dyspepsia!

Where there is early amative excess, especially of an unnatural character, it does not need all this. The less the vital force, the more easily is it exhausted. When a woman's strength is drawn to the uterus, in gestation, her digestion is apt to be feeble. Few have force enough for both processes. The harder any person works, especially in mental labour, the less he should eat. In a tolerably healthy system, this regulates itself, for much excitement of any kind takes away the appetite. Lawyers, clergymen, merchants, artists, and vast numbers of women, exhausted by dress, dissipation, amativeness, maternity, and unhappy domestic relations, have dyspepsia.

The effects of this disease, besides those mentioned as symptoms, are numerous and distressing. There is scarcely any disease that is not produced by it, or greatly aggravated. Skin diseases of all kinds, ulcers, cough, headache, asthma, functional disease of the heart, uterine diseases, rheumatism and gout, and a host of affections, are the results of this central cause. A depravation of the blood cannot fail to affect every organ, every secretion, every process, every function of the body. Whatever the disease, if we find it complicated with dyspepsia, that must be cured, and generally this is sufficient. Cure the dyspepsia, and we cure all that depends upon it.

But how? First by a removal of every cause; and second, by living in the conditions of health. "Cease to do evil—learn to do well." If people who believe the Bible only knew a little of its meaning!

The first requisite in treatment is rest for the poor disordered stomach. The dyspeptic must stop eating. I have already referred to the case of Mr. Robinson of Nantucket, who for several months weighed out his three ounces of dry unbolted wheat-bread a-day; one ounce for breakfast, one for dinner, and sometimes an ounce and sometimes only half an ounce for supper. This was his only food, and water his only drink. He got well, and strong, and even increased in weight on this diet.

We have had patients who have been even more abstemious. The last bad dyspeptic we had, did not eat three ounces in as many weeks, and would have been better without what she did eat. She was packed and bathed, and drank water when thirsty; she was weak, but less so than one would imagine: but at the end of that time there came a healthy hunger and the power of digestion.

This is the true way to cure dyspepsia. Give up to be cured. Eat nothing. Drink soft water. Be bathed, and rubbed, and packed, as your strength will allow. Take frequent injections if constipated; but fasting generally brings on action of the bowels. The stomach is rested, the whole system is purified. Then comes a clean, healthy appetite, and pure secretions. Now be careful. Begin with the smallest quantity or the best food. Increase it very slowly. This is the hardest point, but victory is before you. Go on step by step, and you build up a new constitution; and after being exhausted and broken down, a poor, miserable dyspeptic at thirty-five or forty, you may live, as Cornaro did, to be a hundred.

This is the way to cure dyspepsia, and every disease of which it is a part, which is four-fifths of all our maladies. Dyspeptic reader, here is the road to health; if you do not choose to travel it, it is no fault of mine. Where there is a will, there is a way; and in this case, the best way is the one I have pointed out to you.

Having done my duty in this central matter of dyspepsia, I shall very briefly notice some other diseases of the digestive organs, all more or less connected with, and dependent upon it.

Sick Headache is a symptom of dyspepsia and narcotisation. Every case may be cured by a careful diet, and the disuse of tea, coffee, or tobacco.

Toothache and caries of the teeth are dyspeptic symptoms. Early loss of teeth is a sign of a weak and scrofulous constitution. Strong, well-set, and enduring teeth are signs of a good constitution and a good digestion. Sugar, acids, etc., are supposed to injure the teeth in childhood. They do not affect them directly but by producing disorder of the stomach. A flesh diet also makes the teeth foul and liable to decay. Many persons, subject to caries and toothache, have found the decay stop and the pain cease, after adopting a vegetable diet, with other healthy conditions, the relative importance of which I have no disposition to undervalue.

When the teeth are in a bad condition, covered with tartar, decaying, aching, there are two things to be done. First, go resolutely to a good, intelligent, honest, faithful dentist. Sit down in his chair; have every tooth pulled that cannot be saved; have every carious spot carefully cut out, and filled with pure gold, and all made clean. Then get a good brush, and with soft water, a little clean soap, and some powdered charcoal, keep them so.

The Gums and Tongue are liable to disease, but those affections, I believe, are always connected with some irregularity of diet, or poisoning, and are to be treated accordingly.

Sore Throat is a very common disorder. We have elongation of the uvula, enlargement and ulceration of the tonsils, and inflammation of the pharynx. This is caused by dyspepsia, or amative excess, or both, and treated accordingly, with frequent washings and garglings of the throat with cold water. Exposure to cold sometimes aggravates these affections, and warm clothing and wearing the beard are remedies.

Inflammation of the Stomach, Acute Gastritis, is caused by poison, as arsenic, corrosive sublimate, etc., or by some peculiarly acrid, indigestible food; sometimes by cold, where the organ is very susceptible. There is acute pain, tenderness on pressure, and vomiting with fever.

Give a tepid water emetic, so as to cleanse the stomach thoroughly; empty the bowels by injections; drink cold water frequently, in moderate quantities, and apply the wet compress and wet-sheet pack, according to the amount of fever. Irritation of the stomach often produces cough at night—stomach cough—which can be relieved instantly by drinking a glass of cold water.

Inflammation of the Bowels is more common than of the stomach. It is either acute or chronic; and each is a severe and dangerous disease.

The symptoms are pain about the navel, fixed and extending over the abdomen, nausea, a sense of heat, dejection and prostration. The patient lies on his back, his knees draw up, and shrinks from pressure. This and the continuousness of the pain distinguishes it from colic. The countenance is anxious, the pulse frequent and tense. Black matter is sometimes both vomited and passed by the bowels. At first there is constipation—afterward diarrhœa, with very offensive discharges. In chronic cases there is constipation alternating with diarrhœa. The strength fails, the flesh wastes, and the patient dies of what is called consumption of the bowels. The mesenteric glands are sometimes involved in the disease, and inflame, harden, and suppurate.

It is easy to see how disease of the stomach and small intestines must interfere with the vital action of these organs: but we can scarcely comprehend the shock to the system, and the suddenness of death which sometimes occur in these cases. I have seen inflammation of the bowels produce coma and death in twenty-four hours in a water cure patient, who was recovering from a bilious remittent fever, who would not obey orders, but would eat everything bad. Finally, he ate half a drum of figs.

The treatment, in these cases, must be prompt and heroic. Empty the stomach, empty the bowels, and apply cold to the whole region of the abdomen, with friction of the extremities. Put on large cold compresses, and change them every five minutes, the colder the better. After the symptoms are relieved, us the wet-sheet pack. Starve and drink water until fully recovered.

Inflammation of the Peritoneum is to be treated in the same manner.

Diarrhœa is cured by fasting, drinking water, cold injections after each passage, the wet bandage, and exciting the action of the skin by friction, wet-sheet, or blanket pack. As soon as the skin acts freely, the morbid action of the bowels ceases.

Chronic Diarrhœa, treat as for dyspepsia, with injections after each passage, and sitz-baths and packs. A series of sweatings in the blanket pack has great power over this affection. Let the morning bath be followed with much friction.

Dysentery is an inflammation of the lower part of the large intestines. It is a violent, dangerous epidemic, and at times seems like a contagious disorder. Flesh-eaters are very liable to this, as to all inflammatory diseases. Bad air and water, low, damp situations, and uncleanly habits, are all causes of this disease. Children are more subject to it than adults.

In this disease, we must fast, drink soft water, take ice-cold injections, cold sitz-baths, wear the wet bandage or compress, and use the wet-sheet pack, or the dry, warm blanket pack, according to the strength of the patient and the re-active power. Chilling the surface may increase the internal congestion. With these means, and a little judgment in applying them, we may save every curable case. It is particularly necessary to open the pores of the skin. In both diarrhœa and dysentery the use of ripe juicy fruits, or fruit juices have a remarkable efficacy.

Colic is of two kinds, nervous or spasmodic, and wind colic. The former is limited to some portion of the bowels, and comes on in more decided paroxysms than the other, in which gases, secreted by a morbid

state of the intestines, or arising from the fermentation
of indigestible food, are the cause of pain.

Thorough cleansing of the bowels by injections is
generally an effectual remedy.   The nervous, and more
purely spasmodic kind, however, is more obstinate, and
requires absolute diet, the half-bath, or thorough packing.   Hot fomentations give relief, but rather favour
future attacks, and should be used sparingly.   Intense
cold overcomes spasm, as well as heat, without being
weakening.

Where there is stoppage of the bowels from mechanical or any other cause, give injections to any
extent, to the amount of two or three quarts even, if
needed, but no cathartic medicine.   If there is intus-
susception, or the stoppage of one of the small intestines
by a fold of another part of the tube, every grain of
cathartic medicine increases the difficulty and hastens
the fatal result.   The best treatment, like that of hernia,
is to find the place of difficulty, as nearly as can be,
and apply ice-water or ice, so as to thoroughly chill the
parts.

Some persons are subject to terrible attacks of pain
from the passage of *gall stones*, and from *gravel* in the
ureters.   I have found nothing so effectual in these
cases, as to cool the parts as thoroughly as possible.
Fold a sheet so as to make several thicknesses, wring
out of ice-water, and apply, rubbing the extremities,
putting hot bricks or bottles to the feet, or wrapping
up well in blankets.   Repeat the cold application as
needed.   This is a good method of treating all violent,
painful, local inflammations.

Hernia may be reduced, in almost every case, by
pouring a stream of very cold water upon the part, until
thoroughly cooled, and then pushing up the bowel.
Snow or pounded ice, may also be used in all these cases.

Cholera is the common, mild, sporadic kind; or the
malignant and epidemic.   Each is characterised by

vomiting, purging, pain, and cramps of the bowels. The latter is more severe and fatal, and determined by a specific and, as yet, unknown cause. The same persons are subject to both kinds; for there are in both the same constitutional causes of exhaustion and irritation.

The treatment is the same in both cases, but proportioned to the intensity of the disease, and the strength of the patient. Cleanse and quiet the stomach by large draughts of tepid water; empty the bowels by injections; give a thorough half-bath, or a rubbing sitz-bath, by letting the patient sit in a tub of moderately cold water, and rubbing the bowels for ten or fifteen minutes. Put a wet bandage around him, cover him up well in bed, and rub the extremities till they are warm. If the symptoms return, repeat the rubbing sitz-bath; or if not so severe, use the wet-sheet pack.

I have seen the hot stimulating treatment tried in Asiatic cholera, and it only hastened the fatal result. Medicines are of no avail; mild cases recover in spite of them; but I feel perfectly certain that fewer persons in this country would have died of cholera if there had not been a doctor in it. The statistics of the disease everywhere point to this conclusion. What are called medicines often kill. I believe they seldom cure.

Cholera Infantum is the fatal disease of weak and scrofulous infants, who are exposed to bad air and unhealthy conditions in a hot climate. It is especially the disease of crowded populations. Among its causes, as given by medical writers, are dentition, improper food in all its varieties, including *the milk of a pregnant mother, or one who uses the means to become so*, want of cleanliness, heat, bad air, etc.

It comes on slowly, with feverishness and general derangement of the whole digestive system, sore mouth, fretfulness, thirst, vomiting, diarrhœa, tenesmus, or painful straining at stools; the abdomen is tender, the

T

face haggard, the limbs emaciated; sometimes incessant crying, tossing of arms, and drawing up the feet; in others there is insensibility, approaching to coma. It may carry off a child in one day; or, where not hastened by medicines, may last three months. Every summer, during the hot season, hundreds of children die in New York, every week, of this fatal disease.

Prevention is better than cure; and the two indispensable means for either are good air and good food. Change of air alone is often sufficient for a cure. If we secure a patient good air, and give it very little food, and that of undoubted purity; if we bathe the skin, and wrap the bowels in wet bandages; if we give the wet-sheet pack as often as there is fever, and a cooling injection after each movement of the bowels, it is all we can do, and offers the best promise of cure; but a scrofulous child may dissolve and die, with all our efforts.

Worms.—No healthy child, living in healthy conditions, ever suffered from worms. It may be doubtful whether we should have any of these parasites in a perfectly natural condition; but I am sure that the kinds and quantities that do mischief are the result of disease. For the ordinary kinds of worms, I would use nothing but the common conditions of health, treating symptoms as they appeared, giving coarse bread, grits, and fruit, and frequent injections of cold water to the bowels. If I had a tape-worm, I should try water and starvation; but if this did not answer, I should be much tempted to poison him. Probably the safest way to do this would be to take an ounce or two of spirits of turpentine; a less quantity is more dangerous. A kind of fern is also a good vermifuge. The tape-worm grows to the length of forty or fifty feet, and has a small head, on the sides of which are three suckers, by which he fastens himself to the intestine. Hypoish people, who are simply dyspeptic, are always imagining that they have tape-worm, or some "live critter in their inards." The only certain sign of a tape-worm is to have a few feet or yards of it come away. They come from eating the flesh of pigs, sheep, or cattle, which contain their germs.

Many affections of children, such as bad breath, restlessness, picking the nose, fever, startings, and convulsions, are attributed to worms. These are signs of irritation of the stomach or intestines from *any* cause, and worms is the least likely. Even when worms exist, they are not so apt to be the cause of these bad symptoms as improper food, or too much of even the best that can be eaten. Mince pie, raisins, candy, and green apples are worse than worms.

Liver Complaint.—I can remember when every sick person had liver complaint, and ᵀ can well believe it, for this organ must be affected ᵢ . any unnatural condition of the diet and digestion, or any exhaustion of the system. A large part of all we swallow goes through the liver, and this viscus cannot fail to be often disordered.

The liver is subject to acute inflammation, chronic inflammation, enlargement, shrinking, hardening, softening, excitement, and torpidity. Acute inflammation, marked by pain, tenderness, fever, cough, is to be treated like other inflammations—the other affections like dyspepsia, with the wet compress over the affected region.

Jaundice is cured by the wet-sheet pack and genera treatment, as for dyspepsia.

Constipation is pre-eminently a disease of exhaustion. It is caused by anything that uses up the vital power; by indolence, by licentiousness, by gluttony, and is promoted by inattention to the calls of nature. Habit governs somewhat in this act as in other processes. Food of a too concentrated, fine, and purely nutritious character favours constipation. On the other hand, coarse food, as unbolted wheat, vegetables, and fruits, gives the bowels tone and action.

Constipation is a symptom in many diseases, and a cause of many more. That is, this is one of the chain of causes and effects united. But no cause of constipation is more frequent than the use of purgative medicines.

We cure constipation by the restoration of health. We promote the action of the bowels by proper food, in proper quantities. We relieve, as well as cure, by daily full injections of cold water, by which we cleanse and strengthen. For this purpose the water may be retained fifteen minutes with advantage. If absorbed, it will be because it is needed in the blood. The regular use of the sitz-bath and abdominal bandage, are among the best applications. Perhaps the best of all is the daily use of the fountain bath or rising douche, which acts with great energy on the lower bowel.

Piles are caused by constipation and all its causes; but more especially by sedentary employments and amativeness. They are cured by continence, exercise, and the same remedies as for constipation. The fountain bath, which may now be had portable, in every house, acts like a charm on this painful malady.

Disease of the Heart has been at times a sort of fashion. The action of the heart is liable to derangement in all diseases of exhaustion, but its serious organic affections are very rare. It is an organ remarkably well able to take care of itself. Its possible organic diseases are hypertrophy, or thickening of one or both ventricles, dilatation, and ossification of the valves. These may be indicated by the force or weakness of action, and by certain sounds. Hypertrophy of the right ventricle may cause hemorrhage of the lungs; of the left, apoplexy. All that we can do for a patient in any case, is to give him the best conditions of health, and enjoin the strictest "temperance in all things."

Angina pectoris is a painful, spasmodic, paroxysmal disease of the heart, of the most distressing character. It is rare, and we know little of its cause or cure.

Functional Disorders of the Heart depend upon passional excitements, amative excesses, dyspepsia, hysteria, or exhaustions of any kind, and must be treated accordingly.

The Arteries are liable to inflammation, and to aneurism, a distention which increases till it bursts and causes a fatal hemorrhage. Rare; treated like organic disease of the heart, or, if it can be reached, life may be saved by surgery.

The Veins are also liable to inflammation and distention. Cooling treatment, as the wet-sheet pack, is adapted to one, invigorating to the other.

Dropsies are unabsorbed effusions of serous or watery matter, in serous membranes, morbid cysts, or in the areolar tissue; generally, diseases of exhaustion, and formerly often caused by bleeding. Dropsy sometimes arises from pressure on the large veins, by preventing the return of blood to the heart. In a healthy state of the system, this watery matter is continually poured out of the arteries, and taken up by the veins, exuded, and re-absorbed by the serous membranes.

Hydrocephalus is dropsy of the brain, a fatal disease of infancy and childhood. It is acute or chronic. In the latter case, the head is sometimes enormously enlarged. Its signs are, in the acute kind, vomiting, restlessness, pain in the head—then coma, slight convulsions, strabismus. Then comes a remission of the symptoms, then collapse, and death.

There is dropsy of the pleura and pericardium in the chest.

In the abdomen we have *ascites*, or general effusion from the peritoneum; or encysted dropsy around the liver, or of the ovaries.

Over the whole body, but especially in the lower

extremities, there may be edema or anasarca, dropsy of the flesh or areolar tissue. This occurs in consumption, or from pressure or exhaustion.

Dropsy of the brain is nearly hopeless; that of the heart almost as bad; the pleura re-absorbs more readily; ascites is sometimes cured; encysted dropsy yields to tapping, occasionally; and edema ceases when its special cause has disappeared. On the whole, the prognosis is unfavourable. If there is a capital stock of vitality, we may so invigorate the system, as to promote absorption anywhere. The treatment is to invigorate the system, promote the circulation, and especially strengthen the skin. I have seen a course of alternate wet-sheet and blanket packings do wonders.

Diabetes is a large flow of urine, of either a natural or morbid character. In the latter case it contains sugar formed by some unnatural state of the digestive function. It is curable, in either case, by strict vegetable diet, and the wet-sheet and blanket pack, with other general hygienic regulations. Cases that have resisted the *elite* of the medical profession have yielded to this treatment.

Cancer is concentration of morbid matter and action —of intense malignancy. I believe it to be a constitutional disease, and often hereditary. It attacks the breast and uterus in women, the testicles in men, and the tongue, rectum, stomach, etc., in both sexes. Surgical operations are seldom effectual. I know of but one cure—the strictest diet, verging on starvation —the purest and most invigorating life, and a course of the most active purification. By this means the disease has been in many cases suspended. In this alone is there a well-founded hope of cure.

Stone and Gravel are caused by drinking hard water, by a flesh diet, and by dyspepsia. Soft water, and a fruit diet may effect a cure; but where the stone is large there must be an operation.

Rickets yield to the cold bath, good air, and a pure diet. A wet bandage, and the wet-sheet pack, by relieving the system of scrofula, will expedite the cure. An infant with rickets should be weaned, or have a healthy nurse.

Marasmus, or atrophy, is the last stage of consumption, either of the lungs, the bowels, the spine, or the lacteal glands.

CHAPTER XXI.

DISEASES OF THE GENERATIVE SYSTEM.

EVERY function, when itself in healthy action, is a fountain of life and energy to all the rest of the system. Thus the healthy soul gives strength and beauty to the body; thus the brain showers down its energy upon the organic system; thus the organic system nourishes all the organs of animal life; and in the same way the generative powers give force, and spirit, and intense vigour to every organ of the body and every passion of the soul. It is like the mutual interpenetration and influence of the elements of nature. The water dissolves earth and atmosphere; the air contains vapour of water, telluric emanations, and vegetable and animal aromas; the earth is penetrated by water and air, and all are pervaded by the active forces of heat, electricity, etc.

But when our function is diseased, it brings pain, disorder, and weakness to every other. Poison the brain, and the whole system reels; let disease attack the stomach or intestines, and life trembles; exhaust or disorder in any way the generative function, and the whole being suffers.

Some of the diseases of the generative system are common to both sexes, some peculiar to each.

Masturbation, or the solitary indulgence of amativeness, I have already spoken of as a cause of disease; but it is none the less truly a disease, or a diseased manifestation. Those who practice it are often even more unfortunate than guilty. Inheriting an access of passional desire, and a peculiar excitability of organism, they fall into this morbid expression of morbid feelings.

There is no reason or conscience to govern a·child not two years old, and many such fall into this habit. Many a child sinks into the grave from the infantile practice of masturbation. In these cases, no doubt, disease is hereditary. A diseased parent has impressed the full force of his sensual passions upon his child. A mother has marked her infant with this vice, by having her own amativeness excited during the sacred period of gestation.

This is not always the cause--at least, it is not the sole cause of the disease. In little girls it may come by the accident of some uncleanliness, or eruption, irritating the parts, and compelling the friction which results in the unnatural gratification. Boys are abused by ignorant and libidinous nurses, who play with their organs, both to gratify their own sensuality, and to keep the children quiet or please them, when they are peevish or ill-tempered. Older boys and girls allowed to sleep with servants, or children already corrupted, are initiated into this practice. Children at school, especially at boarding schools, teach each other, and one boy or girl will infect a whole school.

It is said by the highest medical authorities (see Copland's Dictionary), that this practice is fully as common—perhaps more common—with girls than boys. When it is not at first a disease of the generative organs, it soon becomes so. The desire grows by gratification, and the act is accomplished several times a-day.

It is supposed by many that the mischief of this practice is from the loss of semen. The loss of this secretion is certainly exhausting; but this is far from being the greatest source of evil. Boys secrete no semen before puberty, and girls never secrete any. The chief source of mischief is in the nervous orgasm. When prematurely excited, though then imperfect, it gives a shock to the whole system; and when often repeated, the nervous power is greatly exhausted. The vitality of the body goes to supply the immature and exhausted amative organs in the brain and body. The cerebrum is robbed, and the child loses sense and memory; the digestive system is robbed, and we have dyspepsia and decay, with a terrific train of nervous and organic diseases.

Even after the age of puberty, when the organs are fully formed, solitary indulgence is far more exhausting than social. When two persons, loving each other, and adapted to each other, come together in the sexual embrace, nature has provided that a portion of the nervous expenditure of each goes to strengthen the other, and there is much less exhaustion of life. In a union without love, or where all the enjoyment is on one side, the loss is greater. A mere sensual union is destitute of spiritual and magnetic compensation; but where there is the artificial, unnatural excitement of the orgasm, without reciprocity, compensation, or use, the result is only evil.

The following are given by medical writers as among the symptoms or effects of this disease, and cause of diseases:

Loss of memory and mental power; entire concentration of mind and imagination on one feeling and act; a besotted, embarrassed, melancholy, and stupid look; loss of all presence of mind; incapability of bearing the gaze of any one; tremors and apprehensions of future misery; morbid appetite; indigestion and the whole train of dyspeptic symptoms, constipation, fœtid breath, etc.; pale, sallow, cadaverous, or dirty-looking, greasy skin; eruptions of pimples over the face, particularly the forehead, and on the back between the shoulders; hollowness and lack-lustre of the eyes, with a dark circle around them; feebleness of the whole body; indisposition to make any active exertion; weakness, weariness, and dull pain in the small of the back; creeping sensation in the spine. Finally, there comes insanity or idiocy; atrophy, and death by consumption, most probably of the lungs; but often of the spine or the bowels.

"The young girl who gives way to it, loses her colour, grows emaciated, does not increase in proportion to her age; from time to time she complains of pains in the chest, stomach, and back; of lassitude, without there being any known cause to give rise to such symptoms. She grows weak, her pallor increases more and more; her eyes, mouth, her walk, her mode of speaking, all her features, all her carriage, in fact, bespeak languor and indifference. Menstruation comes on, either too much or too little, amid nervous affections, and other serious derangements of health, with which it would not have been accompanied, if the patient had been moral in her conduct; the periods of this evacuation are prolonged or become too frequent, sometimes they are changed into true hemorrhages, and generally are much more in quantity than ordinarily. From this may result, in a longer or shorter period of time, an habitual deranged state of the womb, and consequently a sufficient cause for all the affections or accidents to which this organ is liable. Some solitudinarians have nervous affections, blue devils, pains in the lower abdomen and the whites; their eyes appear sunk; they are encircled with a black ring; sometimes they approach to *strabismus*; the face assumes a sombre aspect, an old and care-worn expression; from weakness they cannot hold themselves upright; they have spinal curvature; they have fever, their hands are almost always damp with perspiration, burning, or else icy cold; in the end they become dry, cracky, trembling, and without power; their arms are characterised by the same peculiarities; the skin is rigid and crepitant; they daily lose that soft and elastic roundness which one feels in touching the skin of persons who enjoy health; they are often also bathed in perspiration during the whole night.

"The teeth of some break; the enamel looks as if it were cracked, or it is broken into small notches like those of a fine saw, results of their close pressure and grinding one against another, occasioned by the convulsions which almost always accompany the acts of solitary indulgence.

"Everything bespeaks in these persons exhaustion, and is indicative of sadness, ennui, and disgust; they are timid; but it is not the amiable timidity of modesty and chastity, which is very different from what they display. The timidity natural to a young person is an ornament to her; theirs overwhelms them; they are more confused than timid; nothing pleases or interests them, neither the society of their relations or companions, nor dancing, nor the occupations of their sex and age. Repose, indolence, and solitude, of which they are at once the sad lovers and victims, alone have charms for them. They not only have no desire for marriage, but an invincible repugnance against it. Numberless pustules sometimes make their appearance, and inscribe, in hideous characters, their passions on their brows, where one would expect to read soft modesty and amiability. They avoid the gaze of visitors, and are embarrassed when one suddenly approaches them."

I copy the quoted paragraphs from a French medical author, who has given this subject great attention, as a warning to youth of both sexes, and especially to parents.

One of the sad, but most natural effects of this habit is the destruction, in a greater or less degree, in both sexes, of the proper action of the generative function. When young men have gone to a certain extent in this practice, they lose the natural desire for women, and even the power of enjoying the pleasures of love. There is either a morbid irritability that produces the orgasm and the loss of semen at the first attempt to penetrate the vagina; or an insensibility that requires unnatural means of excitement; or, finally, an entire impotence, without even the power of erection, when it is required, though it may occur when it is not.

On the other hand, women who have exhausted themselves by secret licentiousness are often so *virtuous* as to hate the sight of a man, and abhor the idea of the holiest expression of mutual love. These are our most censorious prudes, who do not fail to crush and banish from their pure society, any poor girl who yields to the supplications of her lover and her own natural desires.

When a woman so unfortunate is married, she receives the warm embraces of her husband with indifference, and perhaps with disgust or absolute pain. She is cold amid his ecstasies, yields only to his commands, and turns from him with repugnance. Sometimes barrenness is induced, but in most cases nature retains the power of re-production, even when the sense of desire and pleasure is destroyed.

How shall we cure this diseased manifestation, and prevent all these horrible consequences, from which civilisation suffers? Prevention here is the all-important thing. Every man and woman should endeavour to have such a healthy control over their own amative propensities and manifestations, as to avoid giving their children the terrible inheritance of diseased and disordered passions. All nature points out those laws of the passions which man alone, of all beings, and especially civilised man habitually violates.

It is the duty of the parent, the nurse, the teacher, to watch over the child, from its infancy, with the utmost care; to watch for and prevent the first indications of this disease.

Bathing, clothing, bedding, air, food, exercise, every thing should be pure and healthy. In little girls, care should be taken in washing to keep the genital organs free from any cause of irritation. Both girls and boys should be kept from those " evil communications " which " corrupt good manners."

And as soon as the child is old enough to understand any subject whatever, it should be taught by its father or mother the uses and laws of the generative function. Were it possible to keep children in ignorance, where can be the use? But it is not. The animals and the very insects will be their teachers. They will learn enough for evil; but not enough for good. A pure, thorough, scientific knowledge should come from the parent, at an early age, and when the child reposes unlimited confidence in its natural protectors. Thousands of children, of both sexes, are corrupted and ruined from sheer ignorance. The boy who has been instructed in the nature and evils of vice, is warned and armed against it. The girl who understands the physiology of the passions, will neither plunge into solitary debauchery, nor can she be seduced, as the ignorant girl can who falls a victim to some artful man, in a moment of passionate weakness, before she knows what she is doing. Since we are so liable to fall into evils in ignorance, it is better to know them in their consequences, and this knowledge is the safeguard of purity.

But when this habit is formed, and is producing its terrible effects upon the mind and body, how can it be arrested? By moral suasion, combined with hygienic regimen. Not an hour is to be lost in any case where you suspect this evil. Explain lovingly to the child or the youth all the enormity, unnaturalness, and evil consequences of this vice. Encourage him, or her, by every motive of hope and terror, of manhood, virtue, and religion, to overcome it. Provide a pure, simple, and not too nutritious diet, with an avoidance of all exciting food and condiments. Give full employment to mind and body, plenty of exercise in the open air, constant society. There should be no solitude.

In bad cases, where the habit overpowers reason, the patient should never be alone for one moment, night or day. He should only go to bed when so sleepy as to lose himself in a moment. He should rise the moment he wakes. The bed should be hard, with cool and light coverings. A wet bandage may be worn around the loins, and folded so as to cover and protect the genital organs, like a child's diaper. A full cold bath should be taken every morning on rising, and a cool sitz-bath, or the rising douche, on going to bed. Let the bladder be often evacuated, and the bowels kept regular. An injection may be taken on going to bed, with advantage.

If the patient will join in the effort, with a hearty good will, these are the means of cure; if not, he or she should be treated as already insane, and put under any necessary degree of restraint, for loss of the power of will is one of the sad effects of this diseased habit.

The frequent use of the rising douche, or dashing cold water on the genitals, with the free use of the vagina syringe for females, will assist in restoring the tone of the organs.

Society, especially that of proper persons of the opposite sex; reading, in science, history, and biography; the pursuit of such natural studies as botany, mineralogy, and other branches of natural history; the cultivation of music and the arts of design; all that can interest, elevate, and purify the mind, will aid in the cure. On the other hand, everything exciting to voluptuousness and amativeness must be avoided.

Nymphomania in woman, and *Satyriasis* in men, are names given to inflamed and excited conditions of the generative system.   The seats of this disease are in the cerebellum, extending to the whole brain, and involving every feeling; the lower part of the spinal cord, excit-ing continual erections and automatic and spasmodic action; and the generative organs.

Its causes are masturbation; exciting diet; an indo-lent, sensual, and voluptuous life.

The symptoms of this disease are an excessive and perpetual desire for sexual intercourse; a mind filled with lascivious ideas, and excited to frenzy by every voluptuous image ; a real monomania, in which one idea fills the whole horizon to the exclusion of all others. There is no longer any discrimination of beauty, or fitness, or attraction; to the diseased man every female, and even a female animal, is an object of desire. Black or white, old or young, beautiful or ugly, it makes no difference. Under the influence of this disease men have committed rapes on little children and aged women.   It is a frequent cause of incest.

When women or girls are affected with nympho-mania, or furor uterinus, there are similar and even more striking manifestations.   There is often a mild attack at the age of puberty, when girls have such a desire for the other sex, that, as one said, "every man looks like an angel."   They invite familiarity, and seek personal contact under every pretext. Plays and romp-ings are often accompanied with these manifestations. Their embraces are full of warmth—their kisses humid with passion.   When the disease is a little further ad-vanced, they lose all sense of decency; inviting men to sexual commerce by words and gestures, and with pas-sionate tears.   Under these influences women have com-mitted excesses of which men are not capable.   In either sex, this disease may go on to a permanent insanity, and a death as horrible as the imagination can conceive.

The processes of water-cure give us the means of controlling this disease to a remarkable degree. A spare and entirely unstimulating diet, the sitz-bath, the rising douche, the cold douche, or ice-water to the cerebellum, are plainly indicated. The vagina syringe helps to overcome the inflammation of the womb, and the wet bandage, often renewed, should be worn around the loins by women, and should cover the genital organs in men. The treatment is, in fact, very similar to that for masturbation or inflammation of any other part of the system.

Amative diseases and irregularities lead to *Sterility* and *Impotence* in men, and *Barrenness* in women. These are sad afflictions; for nature, with an ever-yearning heart, demands the perpetuation of our species No desire is so universal as that for offspring. It is next to the love of life—often it exceeds it. It pervades the whole organic world, vegetable and animal.

Sterility in men is the result of inaction of the testicles, by which the spermatic animalcules are not produced; or some abnormal condition, which prevents the semen being conveyed to its destination. Exhaustion may stop the secretion. The semen may pass off in involuntary emissions, by night or day, or into the bladder, so as to be voided with the urine; or there may be impotence, or the lack of power to erect the organ, and consummate the sexual act. These conditions may be accompanied with the subsidence of sexual desire, or a state of complete eunuchism; or the desire may exist without the power. Where desire remains, there is more prospect of recovery. Many persons of both sexes are born without amative desire or power.

Masturbation leads directly to impotence in men and women; often to sterility. In women the organs, external and internal, may lose their sensibility to pleasure—there may be merely the cold, indifferent, or even painful or repulsive reception of the masculine embrace, and still the ovaries may form their germs, and the uterus may nourish them. Barrenness in women may proceed from falling or other displacement of the womb; from the closing of its mouth; from leucorrhœa or whites, or other diseased discharge, which may arrest and destroy the zoosperms; or it may be caused by inflammation, or excessive irritability of the uterus, by which the embryos are thrown off in a series of early abortions; and the same result may be produced by the frequent excitement of amativeness and sexual connection in pregnancy.

The cure of sterility in men in those rare cases in which it exists without impotence, must come with health. Use the proper treatment for dyspepsia, or masturbation, or scrofula, or whatever may be the condition of the patient.

The cure of impotence must be a course of gradual invigoration. Put the patient into the best of possible healthy conditions, and the cure will come. As he gains in general vigour, there should be the natural incitements to amativeness. The company and friendly intercourse of strong and affectionate women, the moderate indulgence of the sentiment of voluptuousness, will favour a cure, by gently directing the current of life into the cerebellum, and its special organs.

The impotence of women requires corresponding treatment, with bathing, the sitz-bath, the rising douche, the wet bandage, and the vagina syringe; there should be combined, if possible, the loving magnetism of healthy manhood. This magnetism gives a strength, health, and life, of which few are aware, but which every exhausted nature craves with an infinite longing. When a delicate, exhausted woman lies upon the bosom of a strong man, with his loving arms around her, a new life is infused into her being.

U

But when barrenness comes from excessive action, it must be treated like nymphomania; and the woman who desires to have a child by the man she loves, should receive his embrace at the proper period, which I have already pointed out, and but once. She repeats it at the risk of losing what she most desires. She must wait until the recurrence of the period.

Where there are diseases or displacements, they must be remedied. There are more impotent and sterile men than barren women. Nature has provided for this, in her care for the species. No woman can be the mother of more than twenty or thirty children at the utmost, but any well man might be the father of thousands. A woman can possibly have one or two children every year; a man may possibly have a hundred in the same period.

Among the noblest animals below man, only the most vigorous males are allowed to procreate. Nature has so provided for the conservation of the species; but every miserable, diseased, idiotic specimen of humanity thinks he has a right to beget children, and perpetuate his diseases in a miserable and depraved offspring. There should be some means to prevent the perpetuation of human vices and miseries by hereditary transmission. It cannot be done by Act of Parliament, but I have much faith in the growing intelligence of women, which will teach them the duty of obeying their natural instinct to select the best possible fathers for their children. Women have an unlimited and acknowledged right of rejection, and should firmly exercise it for their own good and the good of their race.

Venereal Diseases are of great importance, since they taint the sources of life, and one of them may affect several generations, and because, in many cases, men, women, and children are the innocent victims to these diseases; and they should have, without needless exposure, the means of cure.   Men give these diseases to their wives, women to their husbands, and children inherit them from one or both parents.

The two diseases, considered venereal, as resulting from a poison communicated by sexual connection, are gonorrhœa and syphilis.

Gonorrhœa has probably existed since men and woman first became diseased.   It is an inflammation of the mucous membrane, caused by a peculiar or specific virus; but this virus may probably be developed at any time, by filthy habits, or by general disease of the constitution.   Thus, if a man have commerce with a woman who has a bad leucorrhœa, or in some cases, during the menstrual period, the result will be a poisoning and inflammation of the urethra, followed by first a mucous and then a purulent discharge.   If the patient is very healthy, he may not take the infection, or may quickly throw it off.   But if his system is full of bad matter, it will be drawn to the diseased surface, and so keep up and increase the discharge.   There may even arise indolent buboes, from the poisoning of the inguinal glands by the matter coming to the part affected, or which is passing off into the system.   If any of this matter comes in contact with the inside of the eyelids, it may produce a gonorrhœal ophthalmia.   The colour of the matter which comes from the urethra is greenish, and this is considered diagnostic of the genuine disease.   In women, this affection exists both in the urethra and the vagina.

It is a filthy and troublesome disease, and even dangerous in some of its results.   When long kept up it causes thickening of the membrane in the male urethra, and consequent stricture, or stoppage of the urine.   It is therefore advisable to adopt at once the means of cure; and especially not to tamper with the remedies so much in vogue, for in this, as in many cases, the disease often has the credit of consequences that belong to the treatment.

A strict diet (and this is of great importance, and in many cases is alone sufficient for rapid cure), bathing the whole body, drinking plentifully of soft water, eating watery fruits, grapes, oranges, melons, etc., and bathing the parts in tepid water, taking tepid sitz-baths, and wrapping in wet cloths, will cure. I say tepid water, because the action of cold may continue and increase the disease. In tender parts and small surfaces, as in gonorrhœa and ophthalmia, it is better not to increase the action of the part by cold.

Women should take many sitz-baths, and use the vagina syringe with tepid water very often. The diet must be very sparing, and contain no greasy or exciting food. So simple is the cure of this disorder.

Syphilis is a virus of a far more malignant kind. It is not known how it was first developed; but there is reason to believe that it has only been known to the civilised world for three centuries. It was not produced by any ordinary debauchery. In the worst days of Babylon or Rome, it was entirely unknown. We find no hint of it in ancient authors, medical, historical, or satirical. It was never described in Europe until the period of the return of Columbus from the discovery of America. In a few years from that time it had spread over Europe, and committed everywhere terrible ravages.

Some have thought that it was developed among the Carib Indians, by the use of the most revolting form of carnivorous diet, the eating of human flesh. Whatever its origin, it soon infected the blood of Spain, spread over Europe, and was carried by commerce to every region of the earth—many of the fairest of which it has depopulated of their original inhabitants. The Europeans who discovered the Eden islands of the Pacific, carried with them two scourges, rum and syphilis. They have since carried them missionaries;

But the aboriginal races will not long remain to enjoy the benefits of their instructions.

There are three forms in which the disease manifests itself. *Primary*, in the chancre, or ulceration of the inoculated part and of glands in its vicinity. This is by the absorption of a concentrated virus of another chancre. *Secondary*, in eating away the cartilages of the throat and nose, and eruptions of the skin. *Tertiary*, in disease of the bones, and general diffusion of the poison through the system.

Each form of the disease may generate its own, or the one more diffused. Thus the primary chancre may re-produce itself in another, or the poison be absorbed and make its appearance in the secondary form. The secondary disease may also produce its own symptoms, or the tertiary. These forms are taken by direct absorption, either from the whole skin, or some particular portion. Thus a person simply sleeping with another, or even in the same bed— possibly by bathing in the same water—may take the disease. The infant with whom it is hereditary, gives it to the nurse, who, in turn, gives it to her husband. We have here no question of moralities; it cannot be said that these persons deserved their disease.

The idea that mercury is a specific in this disease, is now abandoned by a majority of the most enlightened members of the medical profession. On the other hand, it is widely known that the mercurial treatment produces consequences which cannot be distinguished from syphilis. There can be no doubt that there is always a tendency in the system to rid itself of this, as of other poisons, and there is no more doubt that the processes of water-cure are the most powerful, rapid, and successful of all methods by which nature can be assisted in the work of purification.

But in the treatment of this disease we must not forget that we have a real virus to deal with—a poison

of no ordinary kind, one which disorganises where
it goes, until it is either cast out, or loses its force, or
the system becomes habituated to it, as it does to
malaria or other morbific agencies.

The prevention of this disease is a matter of great
importance to individuals and communities. Some
governments have made efforts at its eradication; but
such efforts must be general to be effectual. In many
cities of the continent, prostitutes are registered, and
put under the supervision and protection of the police.
They are obliged to submit to a periodical medical
inspection, and if found diseased, are sent to the
hospital. This makes them careful, and gives a
degree of protection; but the system is seldom carried
out with any thoroughness. The unregistered propagate the disease. In England, a strong opposition to
the contagious diseases acts will probably cause their
repeal. But every philanthropist must admit that
some means should be found to protect innocent
women and children from such contagion.

Women can generally protect themselves if they
wish, by carefully examining the organs of men with
whom they cohabit, and by using the vagina syringe
after every suspicious connection. The examination,
to be thorough, must extend to the glans under the
prepuce and the mouth of the urethra. Men have
scarcely the same means of protection. The ulceration
of the female organs may be at any point from the
labia to the neck of the uterus. A thorough immediate
washing with soap and water lessens the danger of
infection; but the only means of safety which a moral
man can consider, is to never expose himself to the
risk of contagion. When men and women will expose
themselves to this, as to other preventable diseases,
the physician and surgeon must still consider the best
means of cure.

When the parts are in a firm and healthy state, there

will be neither inoculation nor absorption ; and some persons seem to have the power of resisting all kinds of virus. This is a condition of purity and vigour, worthy of the name of health.

The regimen for cure must be the same as in gonorrhœa, but we require more active purifying treatment. I order a wet compress to be kept upon the chancre, frequently changed, and the part to be washed in cold water. It is well to keep up the discharge, and with the alternation of the wet-sheet and blanket pack, to carry off any absorbed matter by the skin. When the hard rim around the ulcer has softened, and its appearance changed to that of a simple ulceration, we may use a dry dressing, or a covering of simple cerate, and let it heal. Most surgeons cut out or burn, with a hot iron or caustic, a sore on its first appearance ; hoping it may have gone no further ; but many doubt its efficacy, believing that the poison is in the circulation before it can produce a sore. After the ulcer is well developed, there is no safety short of thorough treatment for six weeks. In every stage of the disease, we must use the same treatment as for scrofula, or other virulent general diseases, and I have no doubt that a thorough course of water cure treatment will cure every curable case in a shorter period than any other mode of medication, and that it gives a far better chance of a speedy and perfect purification.

Many cases of *Stricture* may be cured by the wet compress, sitz-baths, and careful friction of the part.

Other diseases of the generative organs are to be treated in the same way as corresponding diseases of other organs.

Seminal Emissions demand a few words of very particular notice. Women have no such disease ; but they suffer equally, perhaps, from two causes—profuse menstruation and leucorrhœa.

There are few diseases whose victims are in a more

pitiable condition than those who suffer from seminal losses. The general trouble, loss of semen, and consequent exhaustion, takes place under several different circumstances. In some cases, the seminal loss is attended by a voluptuous dream. Such dreams occur to passionate persons of both sexes. They dream of love, as of other passions, and go on to its consummation, passing through the excitement of sexual connection, and experiencing the orgasm. Waking, the male finds a flow of semen ; the female a quantity of mucus, secreted by the glands of the vagina. Where the action occurs but seldom, and in consequence of the accumulation of vital power in this part of the organism, it may not be a source of any great mischief, and some have supposed it to be a natural mode of relief. I do not so consider it.

In men, in certain states of the system, there comes on an excessive excitability or irritability of the organs, which makes these dreams occur with exhausting frequency. The semen is continually voided, with a ruinous expenditure of nervous power. The seminal vesicles are irritated by the presence of the smallest quantity of the fluid ; the nervous action is excited, and the exhaustion follows. It is difficult for any well man to conceive of the weak, hopeless, miserable, despairing condition of the victim to this disease.

He feels coming upon him all the consequences of masturbation, without having the power to prevent them. The habit is not within his volition. The nervous organism is performing for itself what the voluntary muscles perform for the victim of solitary vice. Hundreds of young men are driven to suicide by this disease—hundreds more drown the sense of suffering by the excesses of dissipation. All hope of a happy domestic life is destroyed. There can be no love, no marriage, no children, no ambition, for all power of mind and body is wasted.

In some cases, the action seems confined to the spinal centre—the cerebellum no longer acts. The semen is voided unconsciously. Sometimes, in extreme cases, it oozes away without erection, or the slightest sensation of pleasure, even passing off with the urine.

He who has carefully read this book thus far, will scarcely need that I should point out the causes of this terrible disease. I will notice a few. Masturbation is the cause in nine cases in ten. When the victim of this diseased habit would stop, he finds that a fiend has taken the place of his volition ; a fiend he has raised, but cannot quell.

All diseasing and debilitating influences may cooperate in causing this condition. Exhaustion, even by natural means, especially in promiscuous or unloving unions, may bring on the irritability of weakness. Married men have it occasionally, as well as single. There is no more potent cause than tobacco ; and the whole class of nervous stimulants favour this action. It is only a particular direction of what we call nervousness. The causes may date back of birth ; and are important to know only that they may be avoided, both for prevention and cure.

In regard to the cure, I have but two or three directions to give besides those given for the cure of masturbation. Let the patient, in all respects, as far as possible place himself in the conditions of health. Let him regulate the quantity of his food by his power of digestion, carefully evacuate his bowels every night, sleep cool, and before going to bed take a sitz-bath, *beginning at a temperature of* 90 *degrees,* and cooling gradually, at the rate of a degree a-day, to moderate the action of the parts, and allay the irritability. Cold water may be applied to the cerebellum. In the morning take a full bath of cold water, and a thorough rubbing. As the cure progresses, the patient

will have his sitz-bath colder, and may apply other
means of invigoration, as dashing cold water upon the
genitals, which may be best done by the fountain bath;
and this may be used at night, but then with the same
precaution of using tepid water at first, and making it
colder by degrees.   When the system has attained to
some degree of vigour, and this diseased action is
conquered, it may be advisable to marry—but it is not
advisable to have children until health is pretty well
established.   There are physicians who, in cases of
seminal loss, prescribe intercourse with some prostitute.
Those who take such prescriptions are likely to find
that the remedy is worse than the disease.

The diseases peculiar to women are so many, of so
frequent occurrence, and of such severity, that half the
time of the medical profession is devoted to their care,
and more than half its revenues depend upon them.
We have libraries of books upon them, special profes-
sorships in our medical colleges, and hosts of doctors,
who give them their exclusive attention.   We have
quack nostrums without number, and instruments of
the most curious and complicated construction.   We
have, moreover, needless and shameless examinations,
with finger and speculum; and libidinous manipula-
tions, to which women and even young girls are subjected, of the most infamous character.   Diseased
women go to doctors, and pay large sums of money
to be felt of, looked into, cauterised or anointed;
when it is all needless, base, mercenary, quackery, or
worse.   Lines of carriages may be seen before the
doors of fashionable surgeons, and their waiting rooms
filled with ladies waiting their turns for their examinations and applications.   The result of all the attention
paid to this subject, all the medicines and instruments
is, that never were diseases of this class so common,
or so incurable in the common practice, as at the
present time.   The books and professors are all at

fault. They have no knowledge of the causes or nature of these diseases, and no idea of their proper treatment. Women are everywhere outraged and abused. When the full chapter of woman's wrongs and sufferings is written, the world will be horrified at the hideous spectacle, and we shall be ashamed of the petty subjects of our fashionable philanthropies.

Amenorrhœa is the technical name given to the *Retention* or *Suppression* of the menses. Retention is where they have never appeared. Suppression, where they stop, after once appearing.

Retention is the consequence of lack of development, or of inaction, of the ovaries, or very rarely of some obstruction, as the closure of the mouth of the womb, or the entrance to the vagina.

Lack of development may occur from hereditary weakness, from scrofula, from any of the causes which hinder the growth of the system. Early exhaustion from masturbation may suspend this development; or the excititation may hasten it into an unhealthy precocity. This depends upon the age at which the practice begins, its degree, and the strength of constitution.

There is much needless alarm and trouble about the simple lack of menstruation. If a girl, at the common age of puberty, is undeveloped, she has but to wait. Give her all healthy conditions, air, exercise, happiness. If she have any symptoms of disease, as indigestion, constipation, or scrofulous affections, give her the treatment prescribed for them.

But are there no means to hasten the development of the generative system? Yes. In her morning bath, let her dash cold water upon her bosom, and wash it thoroughly. Let her wear a wet bandage low around the loins; take one cold sitz-bath a-day, and use the vagina syringe at the morning bath, with the sitz-bath or rising douche on going to bed. A course of gymnastic exercises, with this treatment, and the proper diet and regimen, will do all that art can do in aid of nature.

Retention of the menses from stoppage is indicated by pain and swelling of the abdomen and symptoms like those of pregnancy. Its cure may require a surgical operation.

Suppression is a symptom of some exhaustion, or disease, or new action of the system. Of itself it is of no consequence. What it indicates, may be. It may proceed from inflammation of the ovaries, or womb; from exhaustion, by masturbation or other amative excesses; or from disease of some other organs. It very often occurs when the system is undergoing changes in watercure. There are patients whose menses stop for months, while they are getting purified and strengthened ; and the return of the menses is the sign that these processes are completed. Study, mental excitement, fatigue, local inflammations, fever, cold, debility, and exhaustion, may be causes of suppression, and in every case the cause is to be removed.

The treatment in this case does not differ from that in retention. Give the patient health, and the menses will take care of themselves. Medicines to force menstruation are full of mischief. In any case, the sitz-bath, the wet bandage, and the use of the vagina syringe, will form a part of the treatment. A single use of the fountain bath is better than all medicines. A thorough wet-sheet pack, or blanket pack with a wet bandage about the hips, is one of the best appliances.

Dysmenorrhœa, or painful menstruation, is caused, in many cases, by unnatural or excessive excitement of the organs, or previous exhaustion. There are neuralgic pains in the pelvis; weakness and distress in the small of the back, tenderness of the bosom; the womb is congested; the menstrual secretion is hemorrhage; clots are formed in the uterus, or false membranes, which are expelled with pains and agonies, like those of ordinary childbirth.

During the paroxysms, we have two measures of relief. A long and very cold sitz-bath, or a hot one.   With the hot one, the relief is more immediate, but the cold is best.   When the first symptoms are relieved, the treatment should be commenced in earnest, to prevent their recurrence.   Every possible cause must be abstained from.   Every law of health must be observed.   The local treatment of sitz-baths, or the rising douche, daily increasing in coldness, frictions around the pelvis, the wet bandage, and the vaginal injections must be perseveringly used.   A free, careless, happy unexciting, and unexhausting life, will add much to the efficacy of all measures of relief.   Daily wet-sheet packs, in any bad case, should never be neglected.

Menorrhagia, or profuse menstruation, may be an excessive secretion of the menstrual fluid, or, more commonly, a real hemorrhage.   In a perfectly healthy state, the secretion is light in colour, lasts not over two days, and does not exceed two ounces.   All beyond this is hemorrhage.   In irritated, debilitated, and congested conditions of the ovarian and uterine system, the proper menstrual discharge comes on at irregular intervals, lasts two or three days, and is followed by a week or two of hemorrhage.   In some cases it comes on with perfect regularity, and then lasts, with profuse flooding, for ten days, and does this periodically.

The causes of this disease, whatever they are, must be removed.   Thousands of women are consigned to premature graves; some by the morbid excesses of their own passions, but far more by the sensual and selfish indulgences of those who claim the legal right to murder them in this manner, whom no law of homicide can reach, and upon whose victims no coroner holds an inquest.   Hard and exhausting labour, care, irritation, and anxiety of mind ; neglect, jealousy; these and like hardships, burthens and miseries, cause and aggravate the disease.

During the flooding, quiet, a cool air, and a horizontal position, are usually prescribed. Sometimes the cold wet compress, ice-cold sitz-baths, and injections, will give relief; I have known the douche to act like a charm, falling upon the lower part of the spine. A long wet-sheet pack and the sweating blanket, by deriving to the surface, and equalising the circulation, may cure with magical rapidity. But at other times the heat of the pack seems to increase the flooding. Some get relief from frictions over the pelvic region and the spine by a strong, magnetic, and congenial person; and a pleasurable excitement, an evening party, or a dance, has effected a cure.

Where there are signs of congestion, in the pain and tenderness of the region of the ovaries and uterus, use the dripping sheet, the half-bath, rubbing sitz-bath, and wet-sheet pack. If there is exhaustion, and a lax state of the vessels, give very cold injections, both to the vagina and rectum, and short, often repeated sitz-baths; but all within the re-active power, and not to produce permanent chill. By all means a strict diet; and when one turn is over, persevere in full treatment, to prevent another.

The treatment of this condition will alarm some persons, who think they must not touch cold water during menstruation. In a large practice, extending over many years, and to hundreds of patients, Mrs. Nichols has never directed treatment to be suspended during menstruation; nor has she ever heard of a case where it produced any bad consequences.

Irregular Menstruation may partake of all the preceding conditions, and requires in each case the same treatment.

Inflammation of the Ovaries, characterised by pain, heat, swelling, perhaps redness, in one or both groins,

is to be treated as any other inflammation, by cold compress, bandage, sitz-baths, the wet-sheet pack, with rest,
and a strict diet; or, if severe, absolute diet.

Inflammation of the Womb, the same, with the addition of injections, both to the rectum and vagina, cold,
if they can be borne, or beginning with the chill off.

The ovaries, uterus, and fallopian tubes are so closely
connected in situation and function, that they are generally inflamed together.   The cause may be weakness,
producing determination of some general disturbance,
as cold, or irritation of these organs.   It follows childbirth, abortions, or excessive and violent sexual intercourse.

Prolapsus Uteri—falling of the womb—is the falling
down of that organ, by the weakening of its membraneous supports, and the pressure of the viscera
above, generally increased by tight-lacing, the pressure
of heavy skirts sustained by the abdomen, and adding
to its weight upon the uterus, or by the pressure of a
load of fæces in the constipated rectum, and the daily
efforts to expel them.   These causes, all acting together,
press the uterus down the vagina, until it sometimes
comes out externally.   As nearly all women are exposed
to some of these causes of prolapsus, a large proportion
have more or less of it.   Even young girls, eighteen or
twenty years old, have falling of the womb.   Very few
entirely escape it, for very few women are entirely well.
Whatever exhausts vitality in a woman, may be a cause
of prolapsus uteri.

The cure of prolapsus is to absolutely avoid every
cause.   To live aright; dress aright; refrain from all
causes of exhaustion, and observe every condition of
health.   There is never prolapsus without general debility, and the patient must have general invigoration.
There is seldom prolapsus without many nervous sensations, pain, and a dragging sensation at the small of the
back, bearing down, tenesmus, or painful efforts at stool;

sense of oppression, or goneness at the pit of the stomach, palpitation of the heart, sadness, and low spirits; weakness of the knees; general exhaustion. These sometimes confine the patient to the house, and always greatly interfere with her usefulness and enjoyments.

Prolapsus may be accompanied by *anteversion*, a turning forward, and more rarely *retroversion*, or a turning backward of the uterus. The latter sometimes takes place at an early stage of pregnancy, when the mouth of the uterus presses against the neck of the bladder, while the fundus, or large part, rests against the rectum, and is pressed down by the fæces. In this case the patient must have immediate relief, by drawing off the water in the bladder, and moving the bowels, when the organ will assume its right position. As all displacements depend upon prolapsus, we have only to cure the latter difficulty.

The general treatment for this disease is that which belongs to dyspepsia, or its other complications. It is to be especially invigorating. The local treatment consists of sitz-baths, the frequent use of the vagina syringe, injections twice a-day to the rectum, and a wet bandage of two thicknesses, drawn close around the hips, and pinned so as to support the abdomen. This is the best of supporters, and should be worn constantly, and renewed as often as it is dry or uncomfortable. In prolapsus the fountain bath or rising douche has a very remarkable power and efficacy; and every woman subject to it should have a portable fountain bath in her bed room to use every few hours. This course, with full morning baths, dripping sheets, wet-sheet packs, and a diet more or less strict, according to the degree of dyspepsia, but always simple and almost or quite exclusively vegetable, *will cure.*

In many cases, animal food, even in small quantities, has a direct effect in aggravating uterine diseases.

Ulcerations of the neck of the womb, produced by corroding discharges, and the irritation of continual sexual intercourse, are readily cured by abstinence, general treatment, and vaginal injections of cold water. Cancer of the womb is a determination of cancerous virus, by the same causes. *(See Cancer.)*

Leucorrhœa is the name given to all light-coloured discharges from the vagina, womb, etc., from the simple increase of its mucous secretion, to the most purulent, acrid, and offensive matters. The same general and local treatment as for prolapsus, which it usually accompanies.

Hysteria, or *Hysterics*, is a nervous disease, made up of dyspepsia, uterine, or more properly ovarian disease, and general irritability, consequent upon general exhaustion. Its name signifies a uterine affection, but some men are as hysterical as a woman. Hysterical women suffer cruelly from the idea that when they have hysterics "nothing particular ails them." Poor women! everything ails them. No disease can be more real than this. I copy a description of it from the first medical book I can lay my hands on: "The disorder is generally preceded in its attacks by dejection of spirits, sudden bursts of tears, anxiety of mind, sickness at the stomach, palpitation of the heart, difficulty of breathing, etc. Sometimes there is a shivering over the whole body; a pain is felt in the left side, with a distention advancing upward, till it gets to the stomach, and removing thence into the throat, it causes a sensation as if a ball were lodged there. The disease having now arrived at its height, the patient appears threatened with suffocation, becomes faint, and is affected with stupor and insensibility. The body is now turned backward and forward, the limbs are agitated, and the hands are so firmly closed that it is with difficulty that they can be opened. Wild and irregular actions take place in the alternate fits of laughter, crying, and screaming; incoherent expres-

x

sions are uttered, and occasionally a frothy discharge of
saliva issues from the mouth.   At length the fit abates
—a quantity of wind is expelled upward, with frequent
sighing and sobbing. After the patient appears for some
time quite spent, she recovers the exercise of sense and
motion; but she usually feels a soreness all over the
body, with a severe pain in the head."

Here is a disease of the will; involuntary motions,
not altogether unconscious; a disordered and discordant
state of the nervous system; and a strange jangling of
the animal with the organic. These are not the phenomena of health.   Here are evidences of great passional
and physical disorder.

Chlorosis is the extreme of dyspepsia and amative
exhaustion, with an aggravation of the symptoms of
both.   There is general debility and bloodlessness, with
morbid appetites.

I have no doubt that a fit of hysterics might be relieved
by a thorough cold bath, or dripping sheet, or wet-sheet
pack.   The terror and sympathy of those around the
patient evidently protract and aggravate the fit.   As
hysterical patients are usually impressible, they may be
controlled to a great extent by magnetic influences.

But the great point in these cases is to give strength
to the system, and harmony to all its functions. Wherever the health is deranged, there we must direct our
treatment.   There is dyspepsia always—always uterine
disease, or irritability—always exhaustion of life of
some kind; and usually some passional discordance or
incompatibility.   Treat for these disorders.

In all these diseases of the uterine or ovarian system,
firmly reject the medical treatment in vogue.   There is
not one case in a hundred that requires an examination
per vaginam.   Not one in a thousand that demands the
use of a speculum.   Retroversion of the womb is the
only displacement that ordinarily requires any handling,
and that is of very rare occurrence.

Reject the application of caustic—it was never in-tended for the neck of the uterus; reject pessaries and all instruments to be worn in the vagina—they are foreign substances, and sources of irritation; reject all rattle-traps, and harnesses to be worn outside. When God made woman, he did not forget the muscles and ligaments required for her support. Artificial support diminishes their power. The wet bandage pinned closely round the lower part of the abdomen relieves, strengthens, and supports.

There are, in rare cases, tumors and morbid growths in the uterus, which may call for surgical examinations and operations. Where the symptoms, such as enlarge-ment of the womb, and false signs of pregnancy, point to such affections, employ a good surgeon; never a quack, who is making a fortune out of the misfortunes, diseases, and credulity of women.

CHAPTER XXII.

GESTATION AND PARTURITION.

IT is as natural for a woman to have a child as it is for an apple tree to bear apples, or any animal to bring forth its young. Travellers inform us that when Indian women of North America, in their long marches, find labour approaching, they retire to some quiet place, by the side of a brook, alone, even amid the snows of win-ter, are there delivered, wash the child and themselves in the stream, and join the company again, and the march is delayed but half a.day. This is natural child-birth.

In civilisation, labour usually lasts from six to thirty-six hours, and a woman is kept in bed three or four weeks. Three women die every week, on an average, in the city of New York, from what are called the accidents of childbirth, while more than a thousand children a-year are registered as still-born.

It is even believed by many otherwise intelligent persons, that pain and danger are inseparable from childbirth, by a special edict of the Almighty. Every observer, however, knows the contrary of this; for there are millions of women on the earth, and always have been, whose labours have been safe and easy. I am prepared to show that childbirth is always so, just in proportion as the Laws of Health are obeyed. Just as life is natural, labour is natural; and a natural labour is not a painful or dangerous one.

The organic nerves, with which the uterus is supplied, are never sensitive in a healthy state. It is only in disease that they have pain. No natural process is painful. We might as well suppose that it would be painful to swallow with a healthy pharynx, or to digest with a healthy stomach, as to expel the fœtus with a healthy uterus. All the pain, and difficulty, and danger of childbirth is the result of disease. Banish disease, and we rid ourselves of its consequences.

This is not mere theorising. I testify that I do know. We have had many parturient patients. Some have been attended at their own dwellings; some have remained with us; some have had several children under our care. Just in proportion as these women have been healthy, or have become so, under our treatment, their labours have been easy, and they have recovered quickly from their effects. In several of these cases, where previous labours had been long and severe, they have become short and easy. Under the best circumstances, these labours have not lasted more than fifteen minutes, and have been accomplished with no more than three or four contractions of the uterus, which, in some cases, were very little, and in

others not at all painful.   One patient could not remember, a few hours after, whether she had had any
pain ; another said the efforts were not disagreeable—
she would rather have them than not.   Surely this is
better than to make women dead-drunk on ether or
chloroform !   The question of the use of anesthetics is
one of a choice of evils.   There are cases in which one
may use them.

The question of man-midwifery has been much discussed of late in England and America.   In fact, the
custom of having men to assist women in childbirth is
confined to a recent period of time and a small portion
of even the civilised world.   It was never known elsewhere.   It is a question which I think women should
decide.   If they want men to attend them they should
nave them; and the most proper man is the one a
woman most wants; provided he knows how to give
the requisite assistance.   I hope to give here such
instructions as will enable any man, or any woman, to
do all that is required, in nine hundred and ninety-nine
cases in a thousand.

The first thing to be learned in this matter is to fully
realise what I have stated in the outset, that childbirth
is a *natural process;* and however painful, or complicated, or dangerous it may be made by disease, still
nature must do the work.   Our efforts to assist nature,
to expedite her operations, or to take her own work
out of her hands, generally end in mischief.   The only
cases in which we are justified in interfering is where
her powers are exhausted, or some malformation or
malpresentation renders all her efforts unavailing
These are rare accidents, and always the result of
disease; how rare, even amid all the vices of civilisation, is shown by the following statistics:—

Of twelve thousand six hundred and five deliveries
at the Maternity Hospital in Paris, only one hundred
and seventy-eight required assistance; and instruments

were used in only thirty-seven cases! Yet we have
fashionable doctors, who give ergot, and use the for-
ceps in a large proportion of the cases to which they
are called. The consequences are, prostration, hemorrhage, prolapsus, and long-continued uterine and
general disease. But the common practice of medicine and surgery, discarding all trust in nature, and
relying on drugs and instruments, is full of such hor-
rors, and the world is full of victims. I hope that I
may somewhat diminish the number.

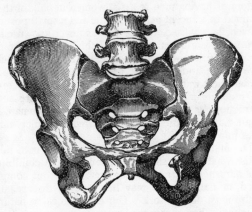

Fig. 45. –The Female Pelvis.

When a woman, fully developed in mind and body,
has that love for some man which makes her desire a
union which will naturally result in the production of
offspring, she owes it to herself, her husband, her child,
and all the possible generations of her posterity, to
prepare herself in the best manner for the enjoyments
of love, and the functions of maternity.

One who is to be a bride, and who hopes to be a
mother should observe all the conditions of health;

and if suffering from any disease, or in the practice of any diseasing habit, she must lose no time in seeking reformation and cure. Let her be calm, temperate, and happy. Let her guard against amative excess. Especially in the honeymoon love runs into absorption and exhaustion; and permanent happiness is sacrificed to a few days of delirious and not very satisfying enjoyment. The tone of the uterine system is relaxed by this excess; the germ is weakened; the spermatic fluid is exhausted of its vital qualities; and the result is a sickly, nervous pregnancy, a protracted and painful parturition, and a sickly, short-lived infant.

When a woman finds herself pregnant, she should double her care and diligence. In this state no strength should be expended in sexual intercourse. "When pregnancy exists," says a distinguished physiologist, "every wish is consummated; satisfied with her work, Nature immediately robs woman of her charms, and of that attraction which brings man toward her."

Every time a husband excites in his wife the sexual passion, he robs his child of some portion of its vitality, and her of some of the strength she needs.

During pregnancy, while a new and powerful action is going on in the uterus—the evolution of a new being—less strength remains to the rest of the system. The stomach has less power of digestion, from which come nausea and vomitings; consequently the food must be more than ever sparing, and of a purer quality. Low spirits and hysterical feelings arise from the limited supply of vital power to the brain. The pregnant woman needs general measures of invigoration; the full morning bath, gentle frictions; the rubbing of the dripping sheet. She needs especially the strength and support of the wet bandage over the abdomen, the derivative action of the cold sitz-bath, and the strengthening effect of the vagina syringe and fountainbath. She may also require, in addition, daily injections to move her bowels. She must take daily exercise in the open air to a moderate extent, but never so as to induce great fatigue; she must live in a cool, pure atmosphere; and sleep, and dress, and eat according to the rules I have so often repeated. Above all, let her diet be pure. Let not the delicate tissues of the unborn child be made up of the flesh of dead animals. The best food of the expectant mother is fruit and vegetables. Too much bread even may supply more bony matter to the fœtus than is favourable to easy birth. And let not its delicate brain and nerves be poisoned with tea, coffee, alcohol, or tobacco, either taken by the mother, herself, or inhaled or absorbed from her husband. Avoid also all the poison of drugs. The fussings and physic, bleedings and dosings which some doctors keep up, during the whole period of pregnancy, cannot but seriously injure both mother and child.

If these directions are followed, there need be no apprehension of the abortion of a healthy fœtus, of miscarriage in the later stage of pregnancy. But some imprudence, excitement, or exhaustion may produce either in a delicate constitution, especially when they have occurred before.

The symptoms of approaching abortion or miscarriage are pain and irregular action in the neighbouring parts, hemorrhage, paroxysms of pain in the back and womb, a feeling of weight, uneasy sensation of the bowels, the descent of the womb, and opening of its mouth. Often these are preceded by signs of the death of the fœtus. These are a sudden cessation of the morning sickness where that exists, or of other sympathetic symptoms as they are called. The breasts become flaccid; the motion of the child, if already perceived, ceases, and a feeling of heaviness takes its place.

Whenever signs of the death of the fœtus show themselves, we must prepare for its expulsion. When there are signs of abortion, and we wish to prevent it, or prepare for it, we use precisely the same treatment. In each case, our effort is to strengthen the nervous power, and the proper action of the uterine system; and what will save the child, when it can be saved, will aid its safe expulsion, when its loss is inevitable.

This treatment consists of cold sitz-baths, and the use of the vagina syringe, the wet bandage, wet-sheet, packs, rest in a reclining or horizontal position, and strict diet, until the danger is over. The expulsion of both fœtus and afterbirth in an early stage of pregnancy require little interference; if in an advanced stage, we proceed, in all respects, as with a common labour.

When the full period of pregnancy has elapsed, and all the usual maternal preparations have been made for the expected, and, it is to be hoped, much wished-for stranger, signs of labour make their appearance.

The uterus contracts itself, and prepares for the grand effort of expulsion. In this way it settles lower down, the abdomen is smaller, and the breathing more free. With this

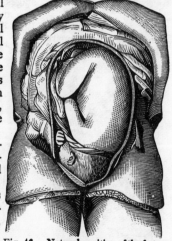

Fig. 46.—Natural position of the fœtus.

there comes such a feeling of strength and lightness to the patient, that if not cautioned, she will start off on some long, exhausting walk, instead of saving her strength. The mouth of the womb begins to dilate, as well as the vagina. There is a disposition to eva-cuate the bladder and rectum with unusual frequency.

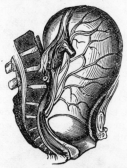

Sometimes there is chill or tremor at the beginning. The preparatory processes are accompanied with the exudation of a glairy mu-cus, provided by nature for the lubrication of the parts, which continues during the whole process.

When the labour is pain-ful, it is divided into two stages—the pains of dilata-tion and those of expulsion. But both processes may take place with little or no pain. At first the efforts

Fig. 47.—Gravid uterus, with the bag of waters protrud-ing into the vagina.

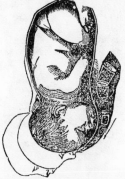

Fig. 48.—Successive posi-tions of the head in the most frequent presentations, the face to the sacrum.

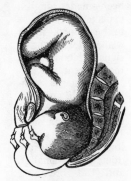

Fig. 49.—Successive posi-tions in birth, when the face presents anteriorly.

occur at long intervals : the pains are in the small of

the back. They are sharp, grinding pains, and seem, as the patient says, to do no good. But after the mouth of the uterus is dilated, the action changes. The body of the uterus contracts with all its fibres, and with wonderful force. This action is quite involuntary, and may occur even after apparent death. But the patient endeavours to assist, and probably does assist the expulsive effort, by holding her breath and bearing down with the muscles of the abdomen.

At first, the membranes, filled with the amnionic fluid, press through the mouth of the uterus, and aid in its expansion. As the pressure increases, the membranes break, and the waters gush out. The uterus, suddenly contracting, seems to gather new force, and the fœtus is pressed rapidly forward.

In a vast majority of cases, we find the head presenting, with the face downward, so that the crown of the head is first born. In a few cases the face is upward, and born first. In very rare cases, the feet or the breech present. In still more rare ones, we may have an arm, or shoulder, or any part of the body.

I will give a careful and exact account of the manner in which I have given professional assistance, in an average case of natural labour; with directions for any probable contingencies. I do this as the best means of instructing others, and in the hope that it may prevent my ever being called upon, except by some one who has personal claims upon me, for a similar service.

When called to a patient, my first object is to establish with her that degree of friendly and familiar confidence which will make my aid agreeable. This is very necessary; and the want of it may make the labour more protracted and severe.

The next point is to ascertain whether labour has commenced; for we have sometimes false alarms, which pass off a fortnight before labour begins. If the pains are irregular, and accompany some disturbance of the bowels, or do not go on with progressive force and rapidity, let the patient take a cold sitz-bath. This will be likely, if they are not labour pains, to send them off entirely. When it is an object to know if labour has begun, it may be ascertained with a considerable degree of certainty by an examination.

I never propose an examination when it can be well avoided; and prefer to wait until the patient demands it, as she does when she grows anxious about the progress of the labour. When necessary to be made, I prefer that the patient lie on her back, with her knees drawn up a little. Then, sitting by the side of the bed, I turn up my cuffs, moisten or oil the forefinger of the hand nearest her, and passing it under the bed-clothes, I carefully and delicately move it along the thigh, separate the labia, pass the finger up the vagina, find the mouth of the uterus, and feel if it is expanded. If the neck of the uterus is quite gone, and its mouth expanded to the size of even a shilling piece, I conclude that labour is well begun. It is best to introduce the finger during a pain, as the patient will bear it better, and to wait until the pain has ceased, the better to find the amount of expansion.

Satisfied that labour has really begun, I see that proper preparations have been made. The room should be cool, airy, and quiet. I prefer but one or two assistants, and should wish never to have a professional nurse, bigoted in the notions of the old school of practice. Any sensible servant or friend, who will follow directions, is better than most of these fussy, important persons. The bed should be hard, and protected from injury by a covering of oil-cloth, India-rubber cloth, or blankets and sheets. I have several towels, a long towel or abdominal bandage, warm water to wash my hands, and cold water to use for injections, etc., a good vagina syringe, which I put in order, so that it will work easily and perfectly fill, a sharp pair of scissors, and two strong ligatures. When everything is in order, and going on properly, if the labour is to last some hours, there is nothing for it but patience. It is impossible to hurry matters—or, if possible, very wrong. Nature takes just as much time as is needful. There is no better economist. It is very likely that she knows how to make a beautiful live baby, and don't know how to "born it." I feel a perfect confidence in her powers, and let my patient see that I do. Generally I can fix the time of birth, and I have done so often within five minutes by the watch. But I am careful not to promise too much.

At an early stage of labour, the bowels should be moved freely, and an opportunity given the patient to urinate often. During the dilating pains, no support can be of much service; but after the regular bearing-down pains have set in, a bandage put around the loins, and held firmly by an assistant standing in front of the patient, at each pain, sometimes is a great relief.

Position is of little consequence. Some ladies like to sit in a chair; some walk about the room, and stand, sit, or kneel at each pain, holding on by whatever is handy; some lie on the side, to be delivered, and some on the back. I had one who preferred to be delivered on her knees, and it proved to be a very convenient way. I prefer that the patient should lie on her back, with her right side toward me. The clothing should be such as not to be in the way, and to be easily removed.

As the pains become more frequent and more severe, the patient and friends grow anxious to know if all is right. I am now compelled to make another examination. If the weather is very warm, I beg leave to remove my coat; but if the room is cool, I ask some one to pin a napkin around my arm; to protect the sleeves. With this precaution, I make an examination during a pain, and find the bag of waters protruding, and by waiting until the pain has passed off, and the pressure is diminished, I am able to distinguish the presenting part; the head, by its hardness and rotundity, or the breech, by its softness and shape. I am able to assure the patient that all is right, if I find it so; and I have seldom found it otherwise in a water-cure patient.

When the increased frequency of the pains and force of the contractions, with sturdy downward efforts on the part of the patient, show that the end is near, I stay by; and when I hear the gush of waters from the breaking of the membranes, I am ready to receive the head of the child. It may not come; but I find at the next effort where it is. Generally it comes down to the external orifice, and nothing is wanted but the dilatation of the perineum.

Now, if the head is large, birth, to one unaccustomed to it, would seem impossible. There is a great bulging tumor, and at the upper part the external orifice of the vagina, nearly as small as ever. If the efforts are very energetic, I involuntarily try to protect the perineum from rupture, by holding my hand so as to restrain a little the forward pressure. There has been much dispute about the use of this, and I have seldom thought it needed; but in some cases I have resorted to it from an apparent necessity.

Suddenly, the head emerges, comes out like a shot, and the patient feels a sensible relief; perhaps a thrill of delight, at the first cry of her child. The whole body may follow at once, or there may be a short pause, and the body, turning sidewise, is expelled by another contraction. The child is born. I lay it on the right side, see that its face is free from any portion of membrane or other hindrance to breathing, that the umbilical cord is not about its neck, and that fresh air comes to it, while I hold the cord between the thumb and finger of the left hand, so as to feel its pulsations. When it has done pulsating, or as soon as the child is crying lustily, I take a ligature, and tie it tightly and firmly an inch and a half from the abdomen. Then another, and tie that an inch further. This last is not absolutely necessary. Then, taking the scissors, and seeing that there are no little toes or fingers in the way, I cut between the ligatures, lay the child on a soft cloth prepared to receive it, and hand it to the nurse.

If there is any delay in the child's breathing after birth, let the cool air come upon its skin, which is the natural excitant of respiration; or blow a sudden puff of air on its face and chest; or sprinkle them with cold water; or wet them. If these do not answer, hold the nose, and inflate the lungs by blowing into the mouth, and then press the air out. This may be kept up for an hour; for children have so been brought to life. In these cases, it is thought best to lay the babe on its right side, to favour the closure of the *foramen ovale.*

Now, or while this was doing, I pass my hand under the clothes upon the abdomen of the mother; to see, first, if there is another child; secondly, if the afterbirth has been expelled from the uterus; and, thirdly, if that organ is contracting as it ought. Often the placenta is thrown at once into the vagina. If so, it may be easily drawn out by a slight traction on the cord, aided by the partial or entire introduction of the hand, beneath it. In any case, as soon as I have ascertained that there is not another child to be delivered, I lay a towel, four-fold, wrung out of cold water, on the abdomen. This assists in the contraction of the uterus, helps to throw off the placenta, if still adherent, and to expel it, and is a safeguard against hemorrhage.

I prefer, if possible, to end the labour at once, by the delivery of the afterbirth, but this must not be done bunglingly, and unless one feels quite sure, it had better not be attempted. It will generally come away in half an hour. When the delivery is complete, I take the vagina syringe and throw a pint and a half of cold water, full and far up the vagina; and if contraction has not taken place, so as to prevent it, into the uterus. This will seem strange and harsh; but in almost every case the patient draws a long breath, and exclaims, "Oh, how good that feels!" Next, the soiled clothes around her are to be removed, and a wet bandage pinned closely around the abdomen. Some give a sitz-bath, but I prefer, just now, the horizontal position, in all delicate cases. Then the patient's clothing is to be removed; she is to be washed all over; have clean clothes put on, be removed to the nice side of the bed, by being carefully lifted over; a wet cloth is to be laid upon the parts with a dry one over it, and the babe given her to nurse. I now leave her to rest and sleep, without eating, directing that, when she wakes, she shall be helped into a sitz-bath by the bedside; sit there five minutes; be washed all over; use the vagina syringe, and have a fresh bandage put around her, and then have some breakfast; a little brown wheat bread toast, or some wheaten porridge, a cup of milk, and a little nice fruit, or something equally good. She is now to take two sitz-baths a-day, one full sponge or towel bath, have the bandage renewed two or three times, and use the vagina syringe at least four times a-day. A tolerably healthy woman will be able to take her baths the third day without assistance; and be round the house in a week, and might even drive out in that time. How many poor women are hard at work when their babies are a week old! Still, when there is no necessity, it is better to keep quiet a little longer.

Such is the best water-cure practice in ordinary childbirth; but we have many cases of women of good constitutions, who have been faithful in their preparatory treatment, whose labours are over in less than an hour, without the least trouble, and who might be round the next day, if they chose, carrying their babies. Water-cure, in fact, brings to women the strength and power of their natural condition. There are women who are shocked at the indelicacy and want of refinement shown in these easy labours; such ought to have the privilege of suffering as much as their sense of delicacy and ideas of refinement require.

There are a few points connected with unnatural labours which require some notice.

When there is a breech presentation, there is usually no difficulty; for the breech and thighs are scarcely as large as the head; but if there is much delay, it is best to bring down the legs, which may be done by passing the hand up in the interval of the pains, seizing the feet, and bringing them down, when the whole body will soon follow. We must now attend to the umbilical cord, and see that it is pulled down, so as not to strain it. When all but the head is delivered, we may bring down the arms, and the head will soon be born.

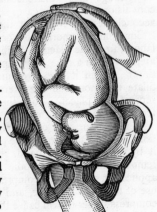

We may even carefully assist in the operation, and if there is delay, we may hasten the uterine contractions by laying a cold, wet cloth on the abdomen.

In all other presentations than those of the head, breech, and feet, we may assist nature by turning the child, and bringing down the feet. No direction is required for this, but the very evident one that they must be brought so as to bend the body of the child forward, and not Fig. 50—The operation of turning. backward.

When the presentation is natural, and the pelvis not

Y

much deformed, it the labour is slow, we have nothing to do but wait. Labours may last twenty-four hours, thirty-six hours, forty-eight hours, and yet mother and child do well. We must trust to nature, and wait. We are not to give medicines, or apply instruments, until nature fails. The patient will seem utterly exhausted; but after resting awhile, the efforts begin again, and seem as strong as ever. She declares that she *must* die; but she does not. No woman dies of the mere effort and pain of labour.

Children are born with their heads mashed out of all shape, by the smallness of the pelvis, but they soon come right again.

There are some cases in which art must interfere—where the pelvis is too small to permit the birth of the child, when the uterus is exhausted, when there is hemorrhage that threatens life, and when there are convulsions. In these cases send for the best surgeon accoucheur to be had; but these cases are very rare.

Sometimes hemorrhage occurs at the beginning of labour, from the placenta being over the mouth of the uterus. Such a case may happen once in a thousand times. When it does, we must, as soon as possible, dilate the mouth of the uterus, introduce the hand, separate the placenta from the womb, bring down the feet, and deliver the child.

When hemorrhage occurs after delivery, from retention or partial adhesion of the placenta, we must deliver it by introducing the hand, guided by the cord, first removing the clots of blood. This operation, with the application of the cold compress to the abdomen, the use of the vagina syringe, and the wet bandage, with a compress under it, will cause the uterus to contract and the hemorrhage to cease.

The signs of internal hemorrhage are great chilliness, bloodless lips, a small, quick pulse, and faintness. The uterus may be felt—a large irregular mass. We shall find it filled with clotted blood and the afterbirth, which must be removed.

It is useless for me to give directions for the use of instruments—I have only to say that they are only to be resorted to in case of imperious necessity to save the life of mother and child, if possible; the mother alone, if there must be a choice; or the child, if the mother cannot be saved. Dr. Dewees, in the course of his practice in Philadelphia, had three thousand labour cases, and was never obliged to destroy the life of a child. One of our fashionable malaperts, in the same practice, would have killed scores.

In all cases of labour of moderate duration, it is better for the patient not to eat, but be content with an occasional draught of water. When all the power of the system is or should be in the uterus the stomach cannot digest. When food has been taken shortly before labour, it is generally vomited.

In summer, if the water at hand is not very cold, we should have ice to cool it, in case of need.

All attempts to dilate the vagina are irritating, and full of mischief, and are only made in good faith by very ignorant persons. Still there are plenty of quacks who sit by the bedside, pretending to "help" the patient. I have known women to be angry, because the accoucheur would not practice this indecent humbug.

When the pains grow slack and irregular, a cold sitz-bath of ten minutes first quite suspends them for a short period, and then causes them to come on strong and regular. In a long labour, a sitz-bath may be given every four or five hours with decided advantage.

Where the external parts dilate slowly, the patient had better be discouraged from all voluntary efforts, leaving the downward pressure entirely to the action of the uterus.

We avoid pulling hard on the navel string, or any forcible extrication of the placenta. for fear of turning the uterus wrong side outward, an accident which has sometimes occurred from much violence, and which, if not remedied at once, by the restoration of the organ to its right position, soon becomes impossible to remedy.

If there is any delay in the expulsion of the placenta, placing the child to the breast is one of the best means of bringing on the necessary contractions.

After-pains never occur in an entirely healthy uterus. They are the efforts at a full contraction, and are sometimes caused or aggravated by portions of the membranes, or clots, remaining in the womb.

A cleansing discharge, called the lochia, is kept up for ten or twelve days after delivery, in the common practice. In that I have given, it is over in four or five.

CHAPTER XXIII.

LACTATION AND THE MANAGEMENT OF INFANTS.

WHEN the nurse takes the infant, it is covered with a slimy matter, with more or less of a whitish substance, not easy to remove. Some babies are much cleaner than others, but all need a pretty thorough washing. The water should be nearly blood-warm ; and it is best to rub the skin all over first with some sweet oil, especially in the folds of the skin. Wash it with some fine, delicate soap and water, taking great care not to get the soap-suds into the eyes.

The next thing is the dressing of the navel string. Take a piece of old, fine, soft linen, fold it so as to make a piece as large as the palm of your hand of four thicknesses, cut a hole through the middle, so as to draw the navel string through it. Put a thin linen bandage over all, to keep it in place.

Now baby is ready to be dressed. Its clothes must be in every respect comfortable; neither tight enough to impede respiration, nor long enough to prevent its kicking about. Its arms and neck should be covered, as well as its legs. The diaper should be loose, so as not to chafe, and pinned with a patent safety pin. Most poor babies are strangled, and fettered, and chilled with their clothes.

A babe wants three things—warmth, food, and sleep; yes, one more, not less important, *love*. Babies not wanted and not loved die in great numbers. It is not to be chilled with cold water or cold air—few civilised babies can bear either. The air it breathes should be cool and pure; but there is no sense in freezing a child. It is best to accustom it to cold by degrees. For the first month let it be washed in water at 80° or 85°, the second it may be 70°, the third 60°, and after that it may take its chance.

Our practice has been to use the cool or cold bath, given quickly, in the morning, for invigoration; and a tepid one at night, with a more thorough washing, for cleanliness. The nurse should be careful to wash all the folds of the skin, and in girls the private parts; and if the skin chafes, use a little sweet oil, or fresh butter, or sweet cream.

A child should have a motion of the bowels soon after birth. If it does not have one within twelve hours, an injection of tepid water should be given, with a little syringe, holding one or two ounces. And whenever, at any time, the bowels do not act regularly, or whenever there are signs of pain in the abdomen, the first thing done should be to give injections until the bowels are moved; and the next, to put around them a cool or cold wet bandage. Rubbing the bowels gently with the hand is also very good.

The navel-string shrivels up and comes off in five or six days. Scrofulous children are liable to have an open or even an ulcerated umbilicus. The application of the wet compress rather increases this action, by exciting the part. It is "too drawing." It is better to dress the part with a rag, covered with a little oil, or simple cerate, made of oil and wax.

Sometimes the breast of the mother is gushing with milk when her child is born; at others, it does not come for hours. Nothing helps more to bring it than the sucking of the child. It may also be promoted by bathing the breasts in cold water, and wearing upon them the wet compress. Let it be remembered that cold water assists action everywhere, while warm water weakens it. If you wish to prevent the flow of milk, bathe in warm water.

Leave the child twenty-four hours to get his breakfast. He will not suffer in that time; but if he does not get any then, it will be necessary to feed him. And the proper artificial food for a new-born infant is two-thirds of pure healthy cow's milk, one-third water, and a very little sugar. This is better than any pap, being a close imitation of the mother's milk.

A diseased or scrofulous woman should not think of nursing her child. And food, prepared as above, is better than the milk of most hired wet nurses. When you find a woman as healthy and with as good habits as a cow, you can let her nurse your child. And it must be remembered that if the nurse has a live baby, *it* also has some of the natural rights of humanity. Every mother ought to nurse her own child, if she is fit to do it, and no woman is fit to have a child who is not fit to nurse it. But our life is in many cases a choice of evils.

How often must an infant nurse or be fed? Some say, as often as they like. Some children nurse all the time they are not asleep. But many children are born with dyspepsia and morbid appetites. Whenever a child vomits, it has taken too much. When a new-born infant is fed, it may take three table-spoonfuls. Once in two hours is often enough the first month, and not in an unlimited quantity either. The second month, once in three hours ; the third, once in four. By the time a child is a year old, it should take its three meals a-day, and never eat between meals. The milk may be warmed, but not boiled. For the first year, a child wants no food but milk. The second, it may have with it a little farinacea—brown wheat-bread, and ripe, pulpy, or sweet, juicy fruit, as grapes, strawberries, raspberries, peaches, apples, pears, etc.

There is no way to secure the perfect health, beauty, and regular development of a child, like entire simplicity and regularity in its diet. It should not know there is an unwholesome dainty in the world. Bread, milk, and fruit, are the food of childhood, and it would be well if, for the first five years, it had no other ; it would be no harm, perhaps, if it never had. I do not object to a reasonable variety of vegetables, after a child has got its full set of teeth ; but to candies, cake, pastry, and other breeders of dyspepsia. Even jams and other artificial sweets should be used in moderation, but naturally sweet fruits are as healthful as they are agreeable.

A child should have its daily exercise in the open air, at least, after it is a month old ; and it should never have its face covered night or day, so that it cannot breathe freely. The lungs and blood of a child need pure air, as well as those of a grown person.

A healthy child has no trouble in teething. When there is any fever, it is easily controlled by diminishing its food, giving it cold water to drink, and putting a wet bandage around it, or packing in the wet sheet pack—moving its bowels, if need be. If the gums are inflamed, rub them with cold water—let it suck a rag dipped in water, or a little bag of ice.

Wean at a year old, or as soon as a child has teeth enough to make a good beginning at mastication. If the mother's health suffers from nursing, it is better to wean earlier.

When the second set of teeth come to replace the first, great care should be taken, in children not entirely healthy, to avoid any disagreeable irregularities, by pulling such of the first set as are loose, so as to make way for the permanent teeth.

Education is a process that begins at birth and goes on till death. Life is a school for the soul's development. Education, in a true sense, is integral development—the strengthening and happy exercise of every power and faculty of body and mind. The stimulation and exercise of a few powers of the mind, to the neglect of all the rest of the system, mental and physical, is a false and mischievous system ; full of evils to the individual and the race.

I have given an idea of what I mean by the true development and life of man. Education should assist that development, and be a training for that life. Our present systems and courses of education, in families, schools, and colleges, correspond to all systems of life in civilisation. The young ladies' boarding-school is no more artificial, false and ridiculous, than the fashionable life in what is called society, for which it is the preparation ; and our colleges are just as well suited to the training of men, as these are to the development of women.

I hope that a time is coming when men and women, from their birth, will have some chance for a free and true development of what is noble in humanity. I have given here my idea of the nature and relations of man. To his social relations I have only alluded ; I hope to be able, at no distant day, to write further upon this branch of my subject ; for a work is yet to be written upon social physiology and social health.

The laws of the Grand Man, Society, are precisely analogous to those of the Individual. And society has its complex and beautiful Anatomy; its wonderful and mysterious Physiology, its terrible Pathology, and its simple and efficient Therapeutics. These are the subjects to which I would willingly devote my future life

---

CHAPTER XXIV.

DEATH AND IMMORTALITY.

THE present human population of the earth is estimated at one thousand, or twelve hundred, millions. The soil of the planet, with proper culture, might sustain five, perhaps ten times its actual population, before reaching the limit to vegetable, and therefore to animal and human life. But for death, the earth would soon be crowded with its inhabitants; and death, no less than life, is the necessary law of nature. If death were to cease, procreation must also cease.

As women usually bear children from the age of twenty to forty, thirty years may be considered the average period of each generation, and this is also about the average length of life in Europe—the higher, or more comfortable classes living a longer—the poorer, and most oppressed, a shorter period. Nearly half of all children die in infancy. In crowded towns, and among the poor, the proportion rises to three-fifths; while the upper classes lose but one-fifth in infancy, and a large proportion live to a good age.

If all men lived natural lives, all would die (accidents

---

* More than twenty years have passed since these words were written, and I have but just published my "HUMAN PHYSIOLOGY THE BASIS OF SANITARY AND SOCIAL SCIENCE!"

excepted) natural deaths. The only natural death is one of gradual decay from old age—the wearing out, or exhaustion, of the vital force. All death by disease, of whatever kind, is unnatural. Our natural life is one of constant, uninterrupted health; our natural death, a painless, gradual decay, and finally a welcome release from a body which can no longer perform its functions as the instrument of the soul. When the uses of the bodily organism have been fully answered, comes the inevitable death. The stock of organic vitality is finally expended. The heart cannot beat on forever, on account of the failure of nervous energy in the centres of organic life.

Of the several periods of human life, some have a limited duration, while others are indefinitely extended. The periods of infancy, childhood, and youth, are marked by striking physical phenomena, and vary but little in their length. It is the same with senility. The failure of the powers of life, when it once begins, is regular and rapid. But there is one stage of existence which may be cut short, or considerably prolonged. This is the period of manhood, or the full perfection of existence. It may last for ten years, or fifty. We know not to what duration it may possibly extend.

In the process of death, we have the reverse of the process of development. First fail the generative functions; next, the animal; lastly, the organic. Still, I believe that each of the former fails, in its turn, from the diminished power of the last. And finally, in the act of death, the system of animal life—of passion, thought, and sensation—dies before the organic system. When the senses have lost their power to feel, when the brain has no longer its consciousness, the chest expands, the heart beats, and the muscles keep up their automatic motions. What we call the agonies of death, are often the unconscious and painless struggles of the organic system, in the midst of which the triumphant soul may be serene and happy, rejoicing in its change to a higher and brighter sphere of existence.

Life has its objects and uses, and premature mortality must therefore be a loss, and a matter of pain and sorrow. The love of life, the instinct of self-preserva tion, the dread of early and unnatural death, are im planted in us by the Creator. But the calm death which follows at the close of a long and well spent life, is the most beautiful thing in our earthly existence.

We must hope for a state of earthly life—a condition of individual development, and social harmony—in which long lives and happy deaths will be the rule, and not the exception ; but, in our present state, an early death is not without its compensations to the one who dies, and its consolations to survivors. If the soul enters the next sphere of existence under certain disadvantages, from the lack of that development and discipline which this earthly life was intended to give, it may also have escaped many depravations. Life, in its present discordant and diseased state, so full of poverties and miseries, offers little temptation to the soul to stay ; still, it is our duty to live out our terms of life ; to battle for the right ; to try to make life for others more endurable ; to work for the great future which God has in store for humanity ; and, in doing this, to enjoy all of happiness that belongs to such a life. I have no right to destroy my bodily organisation. I must use it with economy, and to the best advantage. Whenever death comes, by any unavoidable accident, providentially, or in the course of nature, welcome death !—welcome all spheres of action, and of enjoyment that lie beyond ! So far from death being an evil, in its natural order, the greatest imaginable evil would be not to be permitted to die. Continued earthly existence is an idea almost as repugnant as annihilation.

And a feeling of the unnaturalness, and therefore a

horror, of annihilation, and an instinctive or innate belief in a continued, unending existence, are a part of
human nature. We cling to the earthly life; but much
more strongly do we hold to the assurance of immortality. We cheerfully resign the one, because we cannot lose the other.

Happily, the proofs of a continued existence are
frequent, and of overwhelming force. The earthly
life, and the life of the spirit, are not so widely separated as to deprive us of all communication with those
who have gone before us, where we are soon to follow.
In every age, the disembodied have found means to
manifest to their still embodied friends, the one great
fact of their existence, that the life which now is, may
always be influenced by the consideration of the life
to come; which is the basis of the highest morality.
We can conceive of what men might become were they
once certain that there was no hereafter.

In our own time, during the last twenty years, the
manifestations of spirit existence, and the power of
unseen intelligences over matter, have become more
familiar, and more widely known, perhaps, than at any
former period. Men of science have investigated the
phenomena, men of letters have collected the facts, the
ubiquitous press has given the result to the reading
world,—and there is no longer room for doubt that
death is other than a change to a higher phase of life—
and that many spirits who have lived in the flesh can,
and do give us the most convincing proofs of their
continued existence : thus confirming the one great
central doctrine of every religious faith—the faith in
immortality—and giving to men the highest motives to
a true and good life here, in the hope of a never-end-
ing enjoyment of the life to come.

THE END.

INDEX.

Medicine & Society In America

An Arno Press/New York Times Collection

Alcott, William A. **The Physiology of Marriage.** 1866. New Introduction by Charles E. Rosenberg.

Beard, George M. **American Nervousness:** Its Causes and Consequences. 1881. New Introduction by Charles E. Rosenberg.

Beard, George M. **Sexual Neurasthenia.** 5th edition. 1898.

Beecher, Catharine E. **Letters to the People on Health and Happiness.** 1855.

Blackwell, Elizabeth. **Essays in Medical Sociology.** 1902. Two volumes in one.

Blanton, Wyndham B. **Medicine in Virginia in the Seventeenth Century.** 1930.

Bowditch, Henry I. **Public Hygiene in America.** 1877.

Bowditch, N[athaniel] I. **A History of the Massachusetts General Hospital:** To August 5, 1851. 2nd edition. 1872.

Brill, A. A. **Psychanalysis:** Its Theories and Practical Application. 1913.

Cabot, Richard C. **Social Work:** Essays on the Meeting-Ground of Doctor and Social Worker. 1919.

Cathell, D. W. **The Physician Himself and What He Should Add to His Scientific Acquirements.** 2nd edition. 1882. New Introduction by Charles E. Rosenberg.

The Cholera Bulletin. Conducted by an Association of Physicians. Vol. I: Nos. 1–24. 1832. All published. New Introduction by Charles E. Rosenberg.

Clarke, Edward H. **Sex in Education;** or, A Fair Chance for the Girls. 1873.

Committee on the Costs of Medical Care. **Medical Care for the American People:** The Final Report of The Committee on the Costs of Medical Care, No. 28. [1932].

Currie, William. **An Historical Account of the Climates and Diseases of the United States of America.** 1792.

Davenport, Charles Benedict. **Heredity in Relation to Eugenics.** 1911. New Introduction by Charles E. Rosenberg.

Davis, Michael M. **Paying Your Sickness Bills.** 1931.

Disease and Society in Provincial Massachusetts: Collected Accounts, 1736–1939. 1972.

Earle, Pliny. **The Curability of Insanity:** A Series of Studies. 1887.

Falk, I. S., C. Rufus Rorem, and Martha D. Ring. **The Costs of Medical Care:** A Summary of Investigations on The Economic Aspects of the Prevention and Care of Illness, No. 27. 1933.

Faust, Bernhard C. **Catechism of Health:** For the Use of Schools, and for Domestic Instruction. 1794.

Flexner, Abraham. **Medical Education in the United States and Canada**: A Report to The Carnegie Foundation for the Advancement of Teaching, Bulletin Number Four. 1910.

Gross, Samuel D. **Autobiography of Samuel D. Gross, M.D.,** with Sketches of His Contemporaries. Two volumes. 1887.

Hooker, Worthington. **Physician and Patient**; or, A Practical View of the Mutual Duties, Relations and Interests of the Medical Profession and the Community. 1849.

Howe, S. G. **On the Causes of Idiocy.** 1858.

Jackson, James. **A Memoir of James Jackson, Jr., M.D.** 1835.

Jennings, Samuel K. **The Married Lady's Companion, or Poor Man's Friend.** 2nd edition. 1808.

The Maternal Physician; a Treatise on the Nurture and Management of Infants, from the Birth until Two Years Old. 2nd edition. 1818. New Introduction by Charles E. Rosenberg.

Mathews, Joseph McDowell. **How to Succeed in the Practice of Medicine.** 1905.

McCready, Benjamin W. **On the Influences of Trades, Professions, and Occupations in the United States, in the Production of Disease.** 1943.

Mitchell, S. Weir. **Doctor and Patient.** 1888.

Nichols, T[homas] L. **Esoteric Anthropology:** The Mysteries of Man. [1853].

Origins of Public Health in America: Selected Essays, 1820–1855. 1972.

Osler, Sir William. **The Evolution of Modern Medicine.** 1922.

The Physician and Child-Rearing: Two Guides, 1809–1894. 1972.

Rosen, George. **The Specialization of Medicine:** with Particular Reference to Ophthalmology. 1944.

Royce, Samuel. **Deterioration and Race Education.** 1878.

Rush, Benjamin. **Medical Inquiries and Observations.** Four volumes in two. 4th edition. 1815.

Shattuck, Lemuel, Nathaniel P. Banks, Jr., and Jehiel Abbott. **Report of a General Plan for the Promotion of Public and Personal Health.** Massachusetts Sanitary Commission. 1850.

Smith, Stephen. **Doctor in Medicine** and Other Papers on Professional Subjects. 1872.

Still, Andrew T. **Autobiography of Andrew T. Still,** with a History of the Discovery and Development of the Science of Osteopathy. 1897.

Storer, Horatio Robinson. **The Causation, Course, and Treatment of Reflex Insanity in Women.** 1871.

Sydenstricker, Edgar. **Health and Environment.** 1933.

Thomson, Samuel. **A Narrative, of the Life and Medical Discoveries of Samuel Thomson.** 1822.

Ticknor, Caleb. **The Philosophy of Living;** or, The Way to Enjoy Life and Its Comforts. 1836.

U.S. Sanitary Commission. **The Sanitary Commission of the United States Army:** A Succinct Narrative of Its Works and Purposes. 1864.

White, William A. **The Principles of Mental Hygiene.** 1917.

M